D1631069

PL

Cancer Care Nursing

Commissioning Editor: Ninette Premdas/Mairi McCubbin
Development Editor: Sally Davies/Carole McMurray
Project Manager: Andrew Riley
Designer/Design Direction: Charles Gray/Miles Hitchen
Illustration Manager: Jennifer Rose

Cancer and Palliative Care **Nursing**

A guide for students in practice

Penny Howard BSc(Hons) MRes PGCert Cancer Nursing PGCHE RN
Lecturer, Adult Branch Programme Leader, School of Nursing, Midwifery and Physiotherapy, University of Nottingham, Nottingham, UK

Becky Chady BA(Hons) MA PGCFE RN
Lecturer, Palliative and End of Life Care, School of Nursing, Midwifery and Physiotherapy, University of Nottingham, Nottingham, UK

Series Editor:
Karen Holland BSc(Hons) MSc CertEd SRN
Research Fellow, School of Nursing, University of Salford, Salford, UK

Student Adviser:
Philippa Sharp
Student Nurse, Division of Nursing, University of Nottingham, Nottingham, UK

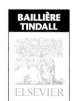

Edinburgh London New York Oxford Philadelphia St Louis Sydney Toronto 2012

BAILLIÈRE
TINDALL
ELSEVIER

ISBN 978-0-7020-4300-0

British Library Cataloguing in Publication Data
A catalogue record for this book is available from the British Library

Library of Congress Cataloging in Publication Data
A catalog record for this book is available from the Library of Congress

Notices
Knowledge and best practice in this field are constantly changing. As new research and experience broaden our understanding, changes in research methods, professional practices, or medical treatment may become necessary.

Practitioners and researchers must always rely on their own experience and knowledge in evaluating and using any information, methods, compounds, or experiments described herein. In using such information or methods they should be mindful of their own safety and the safety of others, including parties for whom they have a professional responsibility.

With respect to any drug or pharmaceutical products identified, readers are advised to check the most current information provided (i) on procedures featured or (ii) by the manufacturer of each product to be administered, to verify the recommended dose or formula, the method and duration of administration, and contraindications. It is the responsibility of practitioners, relying on their own experience and knowledge of their patients, to make diagnoses, to determine dosages and the best treatment for each individual patient, and to take all appropriate safety precautions.

To the fullest extent of the law, neither the Publisher nor the authors, contributors, or editors assume any liability for any injury and/or damage to persons or property as a matter of products liability, negligence or otherwise, or from any use or operation of any methods, products, instructions, or ideas contained in the material herein.

ELSEVIER your source for books, journals and multimedia in the health sciences

www.elsevierhealth.com

Working together to grow
libraries in developing countries

www.elsevier.com | www.bookaid.org | www.sabre.org

ELSEVIER   BOOK AID International   Sabre Foundation

The Publisher's policy is to use **paper manufactured from sustainable forests**

Printed in China

Contents

Section 1
Preparation for practice placement experience 1

Section 2
Placement learning opportunities 77

Contents

Series Preface

Learning to become a nurse is a journey which sees the student engaging in both challenging and life-changing experiences as well as developing their skills and knowledge base in order to be able to practise as a competent and accountable practitioner. To be able to do this requires engagement with others in two different, yet complementary environments, namely the clinical setting and university, with the ultimate aim of learning the necessary knowledge and skills to be able to care for patients, clients and their families in whatever field of practice the student chooses to pursue. The clinical placement becomes the centre of this integrated learning experience.

Tracey Levett-Jones and Sharon Bourgeois (2007) point out, however, that 'there is plenty of evidence, anecdotal and empirical, to suggest that clinical placements can be both tremendous and terrible' but that it is at the same time 'one of the most exciting journeys of your life'. Whilst their book focuses on helping you through this journey in relation to the more 'general' aspects of learning and coping when undertaking your clinical experiences, this series of books sets out to help you gain maximum learning from specific placement-learning opportunities and placements.

The focus of each book is the actual nature of the placements, the client/patient groups you may encounter and the fundamentals of care they might require, together with the evidence-based knowledge and skills that underpin that care. Whilst the general structure of each book might be different, the underpinning principles are the same in each.

To ensure that the learning undertaken in university is linked to that in practice there will be reference to academic regulations, specific learning responsibilities (such as meeting with personal tutors, mentor-student relationships, placement expectations) and the importance of professional accountability.

Each book also outlines how your experiences in practice will help you achieve specific learning outcomes and competencies as specified by the United Kingdom (UK) Nursing and Midwifery Council (NMC). Although the books are primarily aimed at the UK student, the general principles underpinning the care practice described and the underpinning evidence base throughout are valid for all student nurses who are required by their respective international professional organisations to gain experience in a number of clinical environments in order to become competent to practice as a registered qualified nurse.

Nursing is a challenging and rewarding profession. The books in this series offer a foundation of knowledge and learning to support you on your professional journey and their content is based on the editors' and authors' experiences of engaging with students and colleagues in this learning experience. In addition, their content draws on personal experience of working with service users and carers as to what is best practice in caring for people at various stages of life and with various health problems. The ultimate aim is to enable you to use them as 'pocket guides' to learning in a range of clinical placements and specific planned placement learning opportunities, and to share their content with those who manage this learning experience in practice. We hope that you find them a valued resource and companion during your journey to becoming a qualified nurse.

Karen Holland
Series Editor

Student Foreword

Like most students, I have experienced a range of feelings on starting a new placement: the fears and excitement of what experiences you will have, who you are going to meet and work with, what you will learn, and the responsibilities that come with being that bit further along in your training. These are all feelings that are part of our education and training and contribute to the student's growth as a nurse and as an individual. What is expected of you during a placement is another persistent anxiety, in particular, how you can get the best from that specific placement and how you achieve the gold standard of truly incorporating theory into your practice in an effective and useful way.

Most placement experiences vary in length from introductory 2-week placements to full 18-week hub-and-spoke placements. It can take a significant amount of the placement time to settle in, understand the way that particular clinical area works and develop an effective professional relationship with your mentor and other members of staff that enables you to learn and achieve.

This series of books makes the gap between what is taught in the University and practiced in clinical placements much smaller and less frightening. It provides guidance on achieving the Nursing and Midwifery Council (NMC) outcomes and competencies which are essential for becoming a registered nurse, using case studies and real examples to help you. Knowledge of what opportunities to seek in particular clinical areas and how best to achieve them helps considerably, especially when there is so much else to think about. The series also provides a number of opportunities to recap essential knowledge needed for that area (very useful as lectures can seem a long time ago!). From student nurses setting out on that journey to those nearly ending, these books are a valuable resource and support and will help you overcome these sudden panic attacks when you suddenly think 'what do I do now?'. Enjoy them as I have enjoyed being able to have an opportunity to contribute to their development.

Philippa Sharp
3rd Year Student Nurse
University of Nottingham

Introduction

This book is aimed at students who are undertaking a clinical placement identified as specialist cancer/palliative care at any stage of their pre-registration nursing programme. However, the content is transferable to the learning experience for any student nurse who may come into contact with individuals who have cancer, in many diverse healthcare settings. It is also a useful guide for the mentor, in their role of supporting, teaching and assessing students during their practice placement experience. The aim of the book is to equip you with a foundation knowledge of what cancer is, the principles of treatment and the management of symptoms, as well as the nursing care of patients and the support of relatives and carers. In addition, we encourage you to explore your own personal beliefs about, and attitudes to, cancer as an illness and the management of this chronic complex and long term disease.

During your cancer/palliative care placement, you will have the opportunity to meet and care for a wide range of patients; observe complex treatment regimens; work with many multiprofessional team members; learn new knowledge and skills; as well as gain experience and confidence. This book aims to contribute to your preparation for the placement as well as enable you to get the most from the clinical experience. It will also assist in consolidating your theoretical knowledge learnt at university and help you embed this knowledge into your learning in practice, in particular the value and use of an evidence-based approach to care.

Learning may take place within your main placement area ('hub' or 'base'), while other experiences may take place on a shorter placement in another area ('spoke'). At other times, it may be on an insight visit, for instance an afternoon with a nurse specialist or escorting and observing a patient undergoing a procedure. The 'hub and spoke' model of a typical cancer/palliative care placement is fully explained in Section 1, Chapter 7, as an example of a learning pathway. You are also introduced to a range of practitioners and departments within this specialty who will be able to contribute to your learning in practice.

We help you to identify a variety of clinical skills you can learn and become more confident in while on this placement. There are also opportunities identified of how you can gain and develop specific skills for your essential skills clusters, as well as general skills and experience in communication, assessment, nursing handover, discharge planning, referrals to other professionals and participating in a ward round, to name but a few.

The book has an interactive style, assisting you to identify learning opportunities while on placement and to optimise these experiences to meet the learning expectations of your course of study, as well as the generic and field competences required by the NMC competencies. Each section highlights learning opportunities and guides you through a range of activities which generate evidence that can be used to achieve your NMC standards and competencies in the domains of professional values; communication and interpersonal skills; nursing practice and decision making: and leadership, management and team working (NMC 2010).

Nursing and Midwifery Council

Before starting to use this book to support your practice learning, it is important to think about how you might link together learning new knowledge with the outcomes and competencies you are working towards in practice.

As you may be aware from your experiences on your course so far, the NMC is nursing and midwifery's regulatory body in the UK. The NMC is responsible for setting and monitoring standards of work and conduct for nurses and midwives to maintain. Therefore, it acts as a means to help safeguard the public by ensuring the health care delivered by nurses and midwives is high quality.

In order to ensure that nurses are qualifying with the relevant skills and attributes for delivering high standards of person-centred care, the NMC produces standards governing pre-registration education. These standards outline the skills in which nursing students are required to demonstrate that they are competent in order to progress through their course and ultimately register as a qualified nurse. It is these standards which appear as outcomes or competencies for your mentors to sign off in your record of achievement in practice settings. The NMC code (2008) outlines expectations of conduct and performance

for nurses at all times, and compliance with the code is required to maintain safety, high standards and ensure fitness for practice. The NMC has also produced guidance on professional conduct for nursing and midwifery students (NMC 2009). This code outlines the expectations of conduct, behaviour and performance for student nurses while undertaking their pre-registration education. It can be accessed at: http://www.nmc-uk.org/Documents/Guidance/Guidance-on-professional-conduct-for-nursing-and-midwifery-students.pdf

NMC standards for pre-registration education

During the past few years, there have been a number of changes within healthcare and nurse education. In recognition of the changing role of the nurse. The NMC published revised standards for pre-registration education. These govern practice learning for student nurses undertaking pre-registration education on graduate nursing programmes.

The competencies (the term used instead of 'proficiencies') (NMC 2010) are outlined under four domains:
• Domain 1: professional values.
• Domain 2: communication and interpersonal skills.
• Domain 3: nursing practice and decision making.
• Domain 4: leadership, management and team working.

In this book, we only refer to the most recent NMC (2010) standards, domains and competencies. If you commenced your nursing course prior to September 2012 and you are working towards the NMC (2004) education standards, the domains and proficiencies statements will be worded slightly differently. However, there are many similarities and you should be able to see how the materials and activities relate to your own learning outcomes.

How the NMC competencies relate to placement learning in cancer and palliative care nursing

Throughout this book there are plenty of activities and exercises. Alongside each activity we have highlighted which of the four NMC domains and the specific competences the activity relates to, assisting you to build your evidence of clinical experience and enabling you to meet your competency outcomes. For example:

⦿ Reflection Point

Reflect on images about cancer that surround you in society, consider newspapers, TV programmes and conversations. You might talk with other students on your course. What messages are received from the media and other sources regarding cancer as a public health issue? Link your thoughts back to previous practice learning placements and lectures you have had.

Think about why people don't change their behaviour to reduce their personal risk of developing cancer. Consider what your role is as a health promoter.

NMC Domain 1: 1.3; 1.4
NMC Domain 2: 2.6
NMC Domain 3: 3.5

By completing this activity as a piece of evidence, you will gain and develop your knowledge and experience, demonstrating the following domains.

Domain 1: professional values

1.3: All nurses must support and promote the health, wellbeing, rights and dignity of people, groups, communities and populations. These include people whose lives are affected by ill health, disability, ageing, death and dying. Nurses must understand how these activities influence public health.

1.4: All nurses must work in partnership with service users, carers, families, groups, communities and organisations. They must manage risk, and promote health and wellbeing while aiming to empower choices that promote self-care and safety.

Domain 2: communication and interpersonal skills

2.6: All nurses must take every opportunity to encourage health-promoting behaviour through education, role modelling and effective communication.

Domain 3: nursing practice and decision-making

3.5: All nurses must understand public health principles, priorities and practice in order to recognise and respond to the major causes and social determinants of health, illness and health inequalities. They must use a range of information and data to assess the needs of people, groups, communities and populations, and work to improve health, wellbeing and experiences of health care; secure equal access to health screening, health promotion and health care; and promote social inclusion.

This mapping is meant only as a rough guide. There are many learning activities that meet your competencies and you may even consider that some of the suggested activities relate to other competencies (not just the ones listed). As you work through this book and throughout your placements, it will be useful for you to have a copy of the domains handy for completing the work, as well as an exercise book or notebook to record the evidence you start to build up. As you complete an activity, keep a note of the domain and competency. This work can be used as evidence in your portfolio, helping you with your achievement record and to demonstrate competence, whatever stage you are at in your training programme.

See the NMC (2010) standards document for full details of each domain and generic and field-specific competencies: http://standards.nmc-uk.org/PreRegNursing/statutory/competencies/Pages/Competencies.aspx

Sources and evidence

The quality of the portfolio evidence you produce is important in order for you to achieve your competencies, and using supporting literature, policies and research as evidence is key. In contemporary healthcare contexts, nursing practice should be underpinned by evidence. This is outlined in the NMC standards and many policies that govern cancer care. What is classed as evidence can vary depending on the context, it may be health policy or published research. However, evidence can also mean clinical experience, expertise and/or other types of literature. This book acknowledges this broad definition of evidence and, in developing its content, recent research, service users' perspectives, clinical expertise and student experiences have been used as evidence to support, develop and challenge the outline of practice learning in cancer/palliative care placements. Additionally, it highlights the role of a practitioner's (and student's) own values in delivering cancer care alongside these other types of evidence.

We hope that you will find the book helpful while on this particular specialist placement, but also as a guide within any other placement where you will be caring for a patient who has cancer or may require palliative care.

The book is divided into three sections:

Section 1: Preparation for practice placement experience
This section helps you to prepare for your practice placement by introducing some of the theory that will form the foundation of patient care and treatments that you will most likely experience while on your clinical placement.

We focus on the specific cancer/palliative care placement and consider what you might need to know to prepare and make the most of the learning opportunities in order to achieve your learning outcomes and professional competencies.

Section 2: Learning on placement
This section integrates theory into practice, highlighting specific issues involved in caring for patients at all stages of a cancer diagnosis, highlighting specific learning opportunities and activities, enabling you to make the most of your experience and to achieve your learning outcomes and professional competencies.

Section 3: Consolidating learning: the patient experience
In this section, we help you to apply some of the theory to practice by following a patient from pre-diagnosis to after death or survival, in the form of a case study. Your learning is tested by numerous activities (again, all useful towards your competencies) and links back to the theory you cover in Sections 1 and 2. We also encourage you to determine what you have learnt and consolidate your learning by reflecting on your experiences, identifying transferable skills and knowledge to take to other placement areas.

References

Nursing and Midwifery Council, 2004. Standards of proficiency for pre-registration nursing education. NMC, London

Nursing and Midwifery Council, 2008. The code: standards of conduct, performance and ethics for nurses and midwives. NMC, London

Nursing and Midwifery Council, 2009. Guidance on professional conduct for nursing and students. NMC, London

Nursing and Midwifery Council, 2010. Standards for pre-registration education. NMC, London

Section 1. Preparation for practice placement experience

This section focuses on what you need to do and learn about prior to commencing your cancer/palliative care placement.

Chapter 1 explores some of our perceptions and misconceptions of cancer and what shapes our beliefs and ideas about this disease. It then highlights the current significance of cancer and how this impacts on current healthcare provision.

Chapter 2 recaps on normal cell biology and outlines the biological basis of cancer as well as what causes cancer to develop.

Chapter 3 highlights how health promotion strategies, such as cancer awareness, may improve the incidence and mortality rates.

Chapter 4 discusses how cancer is investigated, staged and classified. It also explores the impact of being given a cancer diagnosis.

Chapter 5 introduces a range of definitions used within palliative care nursing to help you prepare for caring for a patient and their family as disease progresses.

Chapter 6 helps you begin to prepare for the learning experience by introducing what might be expected on the placement, what will be expected of you and the skills you will need.

Chapter 7 explains the role of individuals and team members across a range of cancer and palliative care settings, including aspects of health and safety needed in some departments. It also introduces core health and safety information and how to make the most of learning opportunities.

1

Personal and public perceptions of cancer

- To be able to reflect on previous experiences
- To explore what your perception of cancer may be
- To consider the public image of cancer and palliative care
- To understand what the real cancer situation is

Reflection on previous experiences

As you start your preparation for this placement it is important to consider how you are feeling. This can be governed by two key perspectives; the public image of cancer and palliative care and your personal life experiences.

Some of you may have experienced a family member or a friend being diagnosed and treated for cancer. This might mean that this placement is a particularly challenging one for you. Preparation is therefore essential in order to make sense of your feelings and experiences.

Reflecting on our personal and professional experiences can be a good way of understanding what we have encountered. Using a 'model' to guide reflection provides structure and helps to devise an action plan in order to develop practice in the future. Although there are many reflective models available, we have used Driscoll's (2007) reflective model as it is a simple, three-part model that can be adapted to a wide range of situations:

1. What? – returning to the situation.
2. So what? – understanding the feelings.
3. Now what? – thinking about what this means to you.

Reflection point

First think back to 'what' experience you have of knowing a person with cancer.

Now consider 'so what'. How does this make you feel? How has this experience impacted on you and how might it influence you in the future?

The final step is to consider 'now what'

Jot down your thoughts, feelings and actions. Consider what support strategies you have before you begin your placement. This might be something you can discuss with your personal tutor, mentor or a friend on the course. It is very important to talk about cancer with family, friends and colleagues in order to understand feelings and beliefs and to consider what our individual role is as a healthcare professional.

NMC Domain 1: 1.1; 1.8

Writing a reflective account is also an excellent way of demonstrating the NMC competencies. We return to Driscoll's model in Section 3 (see Appendix One) so it is good to start using it early on in your preparations. If you have used and feel confident using another reflective model previously, continue to use it instead.

What your perception of cancer may be

Cancer is a word we are all familiar with and it probably affects most of us in some way, directly or indirectly, but we rarely stop to consider what cancer is. What can we do to reduce the risk of developing cancer? What does a diagnosis of cancer actually mean? This first section helps you prepare for a cancer/palliative care placement by helping you to consider what your pre-existing attitudes and beliefs might be regarding the disease and outcomes. It also refreshes your knowledge and explores possible situations you may encounter, as well as identifying opportunities that might be available.

For many people, cancer is a bewildering disease and often a taboo subject. Some people cannot use the word 'cancer' as it evokes such a range of emotions and thoughts. There are many misunderstandings and assumptions of what cancer is and what causes it. You may have had contact with someone diagnosed with cancer, heard stories about treatment and watched media coverage. As a student, you may have an idea of what you will see and experience while on placement. However, it is important to remember that there are around 200 different types of cancer, each behaving differently (some spreading, some not, some causing death, some not). Each cancer is treated differently and each individual's reaction to the diagnosis of

cancer varies enormously, as does their experience.

Your placement will involve caring for patients who are living or dying with cancer. It is important to remember that patients with cancer do not always die and dying patients do not always have cancer. Much of what you will learn on this cancer/palliative care placement will be transferable to other care settings, as the majority of individuals with cancer are cared for in non-specialist healthcare environments (Gill & Duffy 2010).

> ### (♦) Reflection point
>
> Think about patients with cancer you have cared for in previous placements. How did you feel about this? How did they react? What were their needs? What were your needs?
>
> NMC Domain 1: 1.3
> NMC Domain 4: 4.4

Cancer is a chronic, complex and long-term disease that affects every aspect of an individual's life. Caring for a person and their family starts before diagnosis is given, often in the setting of general practice surgeries and outpatient clinics. Once diagnosis is confirmed, the patient will be under the care of a specialist and may undergo a variety of treatment options which may include surgery, hormone therapy, biological therapy, radiotherapy and chemotherapy.

Even when treatment has been successful and individuals are disease free, patients may be monitored for years, many having to contend with numerous effects of cancer and the consequences of treatment. Alternatively, some may require end of life care. These patient pathways can span over many years or last for just a few days, can take many different routes, pose a range of challenges and bring great rewards.

High-quality and focused nursing care is central to supporting a patient and their family through such an experience and can be incredibly fulfilling. This placement should be a positive experience, and will equip you with essential skills that can be transferred to your next learning placement, into your theoretical work and a variety of assessments. It will result in a better understanding of what cancer is and how it affects patients and families.

The public image of cancer and palliative care

Within the United Kingdom (UK), cancer has a negative connotation often associated with pain, distress, suffering and death. However, the reality is very different and the majority of patients diagnosed with cancer in the UK will lead long and active lives. Some will live with cancer as a chronic disease, others will become disease free and a number will die prematurely from cancer.

Research has advanced our understanding of cancer on the cellular level and of how each type of cancer develops and behaves clinically. Subsequently, there have been developments in diagnostic techniques leading to earlier detection and more accurate staging. There is a wider range of evidence-based treatments available, carefully regulated by the National Institute for Health and Clinical Excellence (NICE).

In an attempt to reduce incidence and mortality rates, cancer has become a prominent focus of health policy. Since the Calman–Hine report (Department of Health (DH) 1995) identified a lack of consistency and the need for specialised cancer services across the country, The NHS Cancer Plan (DH 2000) and The Cancer Reform Strategy (DH 2007, 2008a) have set out specific targets and objectives to improve the prevention, diagnosis, treatment, care and research of cancer. A major focus has been to reduce the delay in diagnosis by improving waiting times, speeding up the time from diagnosis to treatment, improving access to treatment and reducing the number of UK deaths from cancer. The way that cancer healthcare professionals work has changed too. Now working in 'cancer site-specific' multiprofessional teams, decisions regarding treatment and ongoing care are made based on the expert knowledge, experience and collaboration between practitioners, and in partnership with patients. These developments have had a positive effect on survival of patients and their long-term quality of life.

Although survival rates are improving, the incidence of cancer is still rising and there remains a great deal of work to do to improve public health. Having identified some key factors that influence the development of cancer, all healthcare professionals need to consider their role in the prevention of cancer rather than the current National Health service (NHS) focus on managing disease. Two-thirds of cancers could be prevented by simple changes to lifestyle. However, in reality, changing behaviour is not so simple! There are many reasons why people put themselves at risk of developing cancer: lack of knowledge, lack of skill, lack of money and lack of access to healthy living (water, food, shelter, etc.), for example. Consider the undeniable research-based evidence identifying tobacco as a cause of cancer – so why do people still smoke? We need to consider what beliefs and attitudes about the causes and outcomes of cancer people may have. Some believe that 'it won't happen to me' or 'I am going to get it no matter how I behave'. Some do not believe the evidence and may consider that the research is 'propaganda' or feel that 'it's a free country so I can behave however I like'. Many of our beliefs and attitudes are based on those of our parents and family. These become reinforced or challenged by life experiences and by the people around us (friends, colleagues, etc.). The media also play a role by sensationalising research and printing conflicting reports. One day they may report 'Using sun cream reduces the risk of skin cancer'; the following day they may state 'If you use sun cream you'll get rickets'! People are left wondering what the most likely scenario is and have to appraise the evidence, for instance, does it question their behaviour? Which research 'best fits' with their existing beliefs and attitudes? Usually the information least likely to threaten the individual's status quo is the one most likely to be believed and followed.

Many healthcare professionals working in the health service do not see their role encompassing public health and prevention of cancer. However, it is every healthcare worker's responsibility to provide information and guidance and to signpost individuals to appropriate agencies to enable them to make changes to their lifestyle. Not only will this decrease the incidence of cancer, but it should have a positive effect on cardiovascular disease, diabetes and many other life-limiting conditions.

Reflection point

Reflect on images about cancer that surround you in society, and consider newspapers, TV programmes and conversations. You might talk with other students on your course. What messages from the media and other sources regarding cancer as a public health issue? Link your thoughts back to previous practice learning placements and lectures you have had.

Think about why people don't change their behaviour to reduce their personal risk of developing cancer. Consider what your role is as a health promoter.

NMC Domain 1: 1.3; 1.4
NMC Domain 2: 2.6
NMC Domain 3: 3.5

What the real cancer situation is

In the UK, more than one in three people will develop some form of cancer during their lifetime. There are around 298 000 new cases of cancer (excluding non-melanoma skin cancer) diagnosed each year (Cancer Research UK 2010). Over the past 30 years, the incidence of cancer has increased in the UK by 14% in men and 32% in women although, in the last decade, incidence rates have remained fairly constant.

Although there are around 200 different types of cancer, four of them – breast, lung, colorectal and prostate – account for over half (54%) of all new cases. Breast cancer is the most common cancer in the UK with 45 700 new cases in 2007. The incidence of cancer increases with age, with 75% of cases diagnosed in people aged 60 and over, and more than a third of cases in people aged 75 and over. This presents specific challenges as comorbidity may influence the tolerance and acceptability of treatment and the overall outcome. Cancer in children is very rare, accounting for less than 1% of all cases.

Reflection point

Think about the different types of cancer and the ages of individuals that get most media coverage. Do you consider the facts above are presented accurately? Why might this be?

NMC Domain 1: 1.2; 1.3
NMC Domain 3: 3.5

One in four (27%) of all deaths in the UK are due to cancer, more than 156 000 in 2008. Again, lung, bowel, breast and prostate cancer together account for almost a half (47%) of all cancer deaths. More than one in five (22%) of all cancer deaths are from lung cancer, largely due to smoking.

Colorectal cancer is the second most common cause (10%) and breast cancer the third most common cause of cancer death (8%). The good news is that mortality has fallen by 20% in the past 30 years and continues to fall. This is primarily due to earlier detection through screening programmes; better body awareness; improved diagnostic techniques; organisational improvements, such as waiting times; and innovative developments in treatments.

 Activity

Look at the national cancer statistics in more depth on the Cancer Research UK Website, which has lots of up-to-date information on all types of cancer:

http://info.cancerresearchuk.org/cancerstats/index.htm (accessed November 2011).

To look at the cancer incidence and mortality in your specific geographic area, visit the National Cancer Intelligence Network Website which presents and compares regional data from the English cancer registers:

http://www.ncin.org.uk/cancer_information_tools/eatlas.aspx (accessed November 2011).

NMC Domain 1: 1.9

Although the number of people surviving the diagnosis of cancer is improving year on year in the Western world, still a significant number will live with the life-limiting disease, affecting their quality of life and life expectancy. Therefore, it is imperative that the healthcare service provides support and care for this group of patients.

The End of Life Care Strategy (DH 2008b) suggests that, as a nation, we do not talk openly about dying and death, including the needs of people and their family members as they approach the end of life. In addition, relatively few adults talk about their death, tell family members what their choices would be or make funeral plans. The strategy also suggests the healthcare professionals find it difficult to initiate these discussions or help patients plan ahead. This has an impact on planning future care for individuals and can be very distressing for team members. This practice learning placement is an ideal environment to develop skills and competence in talking about advancing disease, patient choices and professional team working.

 Activity

Jot down your thoughts and feelings when you think of the word cancer. Consider how might impact on your preparation for the placement. Feeling anxious? Reflect on why this might be. Now consider who you might talk with about being anxious. Find out if other students in your group are going to the placement area with you. Chatting with people you share experiences with is a great way to feel supported and less anxious.

NMC Domain 1: 1.5; 1.8
NMC Domain 4: 4.4

No matter what the overall outcome, all individuals with cancer require information and support throughout their experience, long after they finish treatment. It is therefore essential that all healthcare professionals are knowledgeable and able to provide this information as and when patients and their families require it. As a student nurse, you are not expected to know everything, but in the future (whatever type of health care you end up working in) you will come across individuals with cancer and should be prepared to answer basic questions. The remaining chapters in this section provide a foundation of knowledge of what cancer is and how the cancer situation can be improved.

References

Cancer Research UK, 2010. CancerStats – cancer statistics for the UK. Cancer Research UK, London. Online. Available at: http://info.cancerresearchuk.org/cancerstats/index.htm (accessed May 2011).

Department of Health, 1995. A policy framework for commissioning cancer services (Calman–Hine report). HMSO, London.

Department of Health, 2000. The NHS cancer plan. HMSO, London.

Department of Health, 2007. The cancer reform strategy. HMSO, London.

Department of Health, 2008a. The cancer reform strategy: maintaining momentum, building for the future – first annual report. HMSO, London.

Department of Health, 2008b. End of life care strategy. HMSO, London.

Driscoll, J., 2007. Practising clinical supervision, 2nd ed. Baillière Tindall, Edinburgh.

Gill, F., Duffy, A., 2010. Caring for cancer patients on non-specialist wards. British Journal of Nursing 19 (12), 761.

Further reading

Bolton, G.E.J., 2010. Reflective practice: writing and professional development, 3rd ed. Sage, London.

Bulman, C., Schutz, S., 2008. Reflective practice in nursing, 4th ed. Wiley–Blackwell, Oxford.

Johns, C., Graham, J., 1996. Using a reflective model of nursing and guided reflection. Nursing Standard 11 (2), 34–38.

Price, B., Harrington, A., 2010. Critical thinking and writing for nursing students. Learning Matters, Exeter.

Websites

Cancer nursing education, videos and other learning materials: http://www.cancernursing.org/ (accessed May 2011).

Department of Health, http://www.dh.gov.uk/en/index.htm (accessed May 2011).

Dying Matters, http://www.dyingmatters.org/ (accessed May 2011).

European Oncology Nursing Society, http://www.cancernurse.eu/ (accessed May 2011).

Macmillan (charity and patient information site), http://www.macmillan.org.uk/Home.aspx (accessed May 2011).

National Cancer Intelligence Network, http://www.ncin.org.uk/cancer_information_tools/eatlas.aspx (accessed May 2011).

National Cancer Intelligence Network, http://www.ncin.org.uk/cancer_information_tools/eatlas.aspx (accessed May 2011).

National Institute for Health and Clinical Excellence, http://www.nice.org.uk/ (accessed May 2011).

National Cancer Institute (USA), http://www.cancer.gov/ (accessed May 2011).

NHS Choices, http://www.nhs.uk/conditions/cancer/Pages/Introduction.aspx (accessed May 2011).

Oncology Nursing Society (USA), http://www.ons.org/ (accessed May 2011).

UK Oncology Nursing Society, http://www.ukons.org/ (accessed May 2011).

2 What cancer is

CHAPTER AIMS

- To understand how cells should work
- To understand what goes wrong to allow a cancer cell to develop
- To understand how cancer cells spread to different parts ot the body
- To understand what causes the DNA to become damaged

Introduction

It is essential that healthcare professionals understand the underlying biological changes that occur during the development of a disease in order to manage the care of an individual. This chapter helps you to understand how and why cancer develops in order for you to identify health promotion strategies to prevent and detect cancer. It also helps you comprehend the principles of cancer treatments, in order to prevent or manage the side effects patients may experience.

Cancer is a term used to refer to a group of diseases. Each of the 200 or so different types of cancer develops for different reasons, will be treated differently and will have a different outcome. Despite this, they all share a common feature – uncontrolled cellular growth.

Cancer is a genetic disease. This does not necessarily mean that it is inherited from our parents, but that it is the consequence of a number of genetic faults in the deoxyribonucleic acid (DNA) in the cell which result in the uncontrollable dividing and reproducing of cells.

How cells should work

A *cell* (Fig. 2.1) is the basic building unit of life. All animal cells are similar in their components, although they may have different functions. Similar cells are grouped together to create *tissues* which carry out specific functions. For example, there are four main types of tissue that make up the human body: muscle, epithelial, nervous and connective tissues.

 Activity

Recall and refresh

Read your biology lecture notes or Waugh and Grant (2010) (see References) or a similar textbook to refresh your memory of the components of a human cell.

NMC Domain 3: 3.2

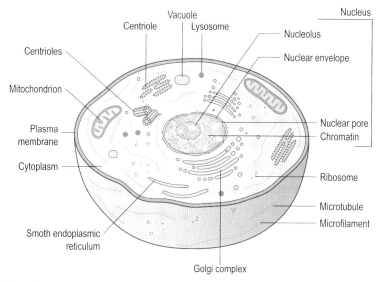

Fig 2.1 The human cell

All cells have the ability to carry out complex tasks, such as the uptake of nutrients and converting this into energy. They are also able to replicate in order to replace damaged or old cells. All the instructions needed to build and maintain the body's functions are contained in the DNA. Each instruction is carried on a unique piece of DNA called a *gene*. Each gene codes for particular proteins which control the function and structure of the individual cell. All the genetic codes make up what is known as the human *genome*. It is a bit like an instruction manual and the genes are chapters in the book with specific information. Genes can be turned on or off depending on the job a cell needs to do.

Each cell contains a complete copy of our genome in the form of 23 separate pairs of *chromosomes* (one set from each of our parents) (Fig. 2.2). For each chromosome and each gene, we have two slightly different copies.

DNA is made up of individual molecules called *nucleotides*, which are in turn made up of a sugar (deoxyribose), a phosphate and a nitrogenous base. The DNA molecule is comprised of two chains of nucleotide bases, arranged in a double helix (Fig. 2.3). There are four bases which are grouped into two types: purines (adenine (A) and guanine (G)) and pyrimidines (thymine (T) and cytosine (C)). Each base is paired up with another base: A pairs with T and C pairs with G. Each base is a slightly different length which gives the double helix its twisted shape. The bases can occur in any sequence. It is the sequence of the bases that makes up the instruction, a bit like the words of an instruction manual. Depending on the sequence of the bases, a particular protein will be produced. The proteins in turn will enable the cell to function in a particular way, including cell replication.

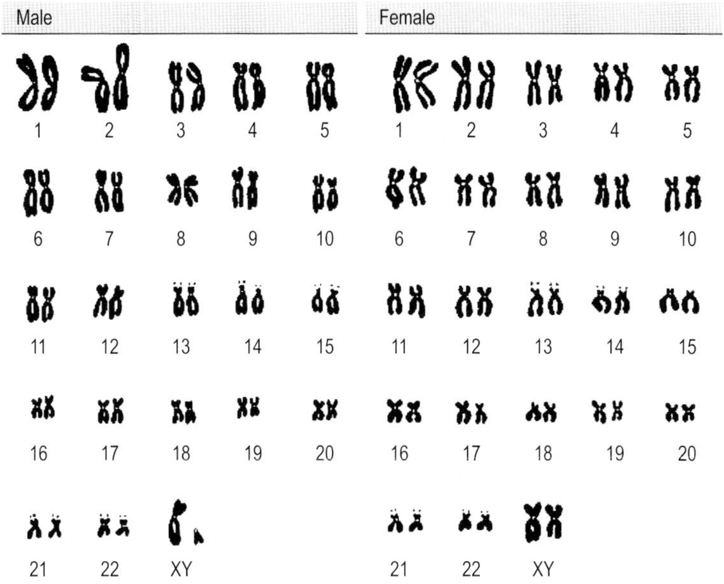

Male						Female				

Fig 2.2 Human chromosomes

Cell cycle

From the time of conception, all of our cells continue to multiply in order for us to grow into an adult. Once we reach adulthood our cells only divide when there is need to repair and replace old damaged cells and to reproduce. To do this, cells go through a process called the *cell cycle* (Fig. 2.4). The phases of the cell cycle are:

- G0: resting phase, not in cell division.
- G1 and G2: the cell builds up energy and prepares for the next stage.
- S: DNA doubles by splitting the double helix.
- M: mitosis where the cell splits into two cells.

By replacing old or damaged cells in a controlled manner, the number of cells in the body remains fairly constant. When cells divide, one cell becomes two. One of these will mature and take on a highly specialised function. The other will rest until it is needed to replicate once again, this is dependent on the cell type. Some cells rarely divide once they are mature; for instance, liver cells divide once every 1 or 2 years. Some cells never divide once they are specialised and are irreplaceable (staying in the G0 phase), such as nerve cells. Some cells can replicate on demand in response to physiological need, for example the endometrium, mammary glands, etc. Others continually replicate, such as blood cells, skin and hair cells, germ cells, bone marrow and the cells lining the stomach (which multiply at least twice a day).

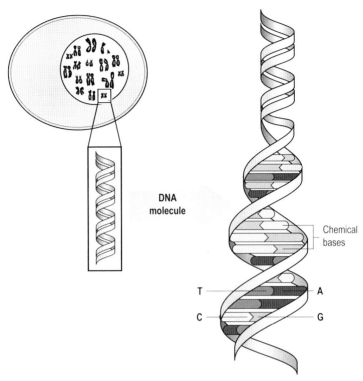

**DNA
molecule**

Chemical
bases

T   A

C   G

Fig 2.3 DNA: the double helix

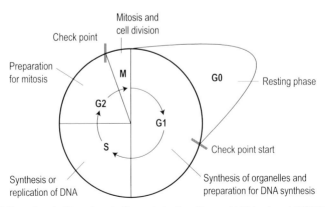

Mitosis and
cell division

Check point

Preparation
for mitosis

M

G0   Resting phase

G2

G1

S

Check point start

Synthesis or
replication of DNA

Synthesis of organelles and
preparation for DNA synthesis

Fig 2.4 The cell cycle. (Reproduced with permission from Kearney N, Richardson A (2005) Nursing patients with cancer: principles and practice. Churchill Livingstone (Fig. 5.4, page 78))

However, all cells have a limited life span, although this varies depending on the cell function and type. Most normal cells divide about 40–60 times before they die of old age. The life span of a cell is controlled by the ends of chromosomes known as *telomeres*. Each time the cell divides, the telomeres get shorter and eventually the cell cannot divide and dies.

Normal cells only divide when they are needed, such as during growth (from conception to adulthood) and to replace old and damaged cells. This replication is carefully controlled by a number of *checkpoints* (see Fig. 2.4), which ensure that cell division only occurs when really necessary and occurs accurately. Certain genes control cell division, known as *proto-oncogenes*. These genes code for proteins and growth factors which signal to the nucleus of the cell to turn the cell cycle on, a bit like an accelerator of a car. There are four main groups of proteins produced by the proto-oncogenes: growth factors, growth factor receptors, signal transducers and nuclear proto-oncogenes and transcription factors.

There are other genes that turn cell division off by coding for proteins that slow everything down, a bit like the brake of a car. These are known as *tumour suppressor genes*. One of the key tumour suppressor genes is known as the 'guardian of the genome' or 'p53'. This controls whether the cell goes into G0 to rest or starts the active cell division process by entering G1. The tumour suppressor genes and the proto-oncogenes work together in order to keep the cell cycle regulated and ensure that cells only divide when they are needed.

During the cell cycle, natural errors occur and the DNA becomes damaged. Normal cells have the ability to repair small amounts of damage by activating *repair genes* which make the necessary corrections. However, if the damage is too great then the cell will destroy itself by committing cell suicide or

apoptosis. This prevents the mutation being passed on to future cells and causing cancer. This may explain why some people might disregard health promotion messages and base their health belief in personal experience: 'My granny smoked 50 a day until she was 95 years old and she didn't develop cancer!' Smoking may well have caused damage to granny's DNA but she may have had very good repair genes or genes that initiated apoptosis, removing the damaged DNA – she did not, therefore, develop cancer.

Unfortunately there is no way of knowing which individuals have mutated or missing repair genes and/or whose cells lack the ability to recognise and to commit cell suicide. Therefore, health promotion is extremely important. We need to prevent or minimise damage to DNA/genes in the first place by healthy lifestyle choices. Second, we need to raise awareness so that people know the signs and symptoms of cancer, ensuring early diagnosis.

What goes wrong to allow a cancer cell to develop?

Cancer is uncontrolled cellular growth which results from the loss of normal regulation of cell division. This is caused by a number of errors/mutations in either a single base (A, T, G or C) in the DNA or a segment of a chromosome. These errors might be a deleted, altered or swapped base. Additionally, a whole segment of a chromosome may not be copied properly or is not repaired or detected and removed by cell suicide.

Although DNA can spontaneously become damaged (which explains why some non-smokers develop lung cancer), generally DNA is altered by an external environmental agent. The error(s) can also be inherited from one or both parents, however this only accounts for 5–10% of all cancers. Remember that we have *two* copies of each gene and even if one copy of a gene gets damaged the other one will continue to control cell division. As we get older and/or are exposed to harmful environmental agents, the second gene may become damaged.

The change in the DNA sequencing results in either less or more or different proteins being produced which then changes the behaviour of the cell.

Since the mapping of the human genome (the entirety of the human hereditary information – length of DNA), a number of genetic mutations resulting in cancer have been identified. This has helped our understanding of how and why cancer develops. For example, 95% of patients with chronic myeloid leukaemia (a type of cancer of the white blood cells – granulocytes) have what is known as a *Philadelphia chromosome*. This occurs when a bit of chromosome 9 swaps with chromosome 22 (9 gets longer and 22 extra short, which is the Philadelphia chromosome). This then codes extra

proteins which in turn increase the production of granulocytes.

Human epidermal receptor 2 (HER2) is another example of a proto-oncogene, which when damaged produces too much protein resulting in breast cells losing control of cell division. HER2 mutation has been found to be present in approximately 30–40% of breast cancers.

It isn't just proto-oncogenes that are affected; approximately 50% of all cancers have a mutated or missing p53 tumour suppressor gene.

One of the key genes which allow the cell to self-destruct (*apoptosis*) is the tumour suppressor gene 'p53'. If p53 is damaged, the cell's ability to kill itself is reduced or lost and the cell can continue to divide unregulated.

Usually there is more than one mutation in the DNA. For instance, many individuals who develop cancer will have mutations in a proto-oncogene (when a proto-oncogene becomes damaged it is known as an

  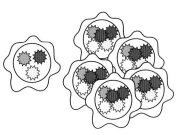

First mutation	**Second mutation**	**Third mutation**	**Further mulitple mutations**
Tumour suppression gene damaged, cells lose ability to stop dividing	Damaged repair gene means that errors are not detected, repair or apoptosis	A proto-oncogene becomes damaged (becoming an oncogene) and cell continually divides	

Time

Fig 2.5 The progression of cancer growth

oncogene), a tumour suppressor gene and a repair gene. These errors will code for different proteins and subsequently the cell will behave differently and cell cycle regulation may be overridden, resulting in uncontrolled growth (Fig. 2.5).

Normal cells divide at different rates, as do cancer cells. The rate of growth of a cancer depends on the cell *'doubling time'*. This is the time it takes for a cell to complete the cell cycle. The time varies from hours to months. For instance, leukaemia (cancer of the white blood cells) may divide very quickly in a matter of hours, and colorectal cancer may divide slowly over approximately 120 days. This has implications for diagnosis and treatment.

There are several other key changes in a cancer cell:

- *Growth*: instead of the telomeres shortening each time the cell divides, cancer cells produce an enzyme called *telomerase* which prevents the shortening and extends the life of the cell.
- *Differentiation*: this is the process where cells mature and become specialised in their function and form. This is a bit like student nurses who, once they become qualified, specialise in cardiac or theatre or cancer nursing. Cells develop a unique function such as a heart or muscle or skin or nerve cell and each is specialised. Usually, the more specialised the cell, the more likely it spends more time in the G0 phase of the cell cycle. Cancer cells lose their differentiation as they become more and more mutated each time they divide. In doing so, they lose their intended function and behave in an inappropriate manner.
- *Tumour heterogeneity*: as a cancer grows and becomes advanced, the cells become more and more mutated, becoming different from one another. This is why some patients do not respond to treatment – some cells are killed, but others survive.
- *Metastatic spread*: a common feature of cancer is its ability to move from one part of the body to another site (often to a distant site). This is known as *metastatic spread*, sometimes known as *secondary disease*. Cancer cells are determined to survive and, once they have outgrown their blood, oxygen and nutrient supply, they will seek a new home that will provide all that they need.

A primary cancer rarely causes a patient to die. It is usually the metastatic disease that causes death and is the most frequent cause of cancer treatment failure. This is because the cells that manage to move and settle somewhere else in the body are usually more mutated and aggressive. Even if 99.9% of cells are killed in a clinically palpable tumour ($=1$ billion cells), a significant number of non-responsive cells remain to continue growing and developing. They are more likely to behave and look differently to each other and normal cells.

Patients often misunderstand secondary or metastatic disease, often thinking that they have a second primary cancer. For instance, a patient with colorectal cancer may think that she/he now has liver cancer as well as colorectal cancer, when in fact they have *colorectal cancer with liver metastases*. It is important to explain the difference between primary and secondary disease as this will affect the treatment plan. Treatment will be selected according to the primary disease, so the patient with colorectal cancer with liver metastases will receive chemotherapy for colorectal cancer, not chemotherapy for liver cancer. This is because the cells from the colorectal region have travelled and settled in the liver, but they remain colorectal cells, however mutated they may become.

Not all cancers metastasise. For instance, glioma and basal cell carcinoma stay at the *primary* site (original anatomical site). Other cancers metastasise very soon after the initial DNA damage, for instance small cell lung cancer.

Approximately 60% of patients will have metastatic disease when they present initially. Of these, 30% will have metastatic disease that will be detected by investigations (such as scans) and the remaining 30% will have microscopic metastatic disease that cannot be detected even using modern technology.

How cancer cells spread to other parts of the body?

It is incredible that cancer cells manage to metastasise as they have to get into the blood stream or lymphatic system to achieve this. They achieve it by developing their own blood supply in a process known as *angiogenesis* or *neovascularisation* and secrete enzymes that dissolve the extracellular matrix. When entering the circulation system, cancer cells have to contend with the body's immune system and very turbulent conditions in blood vessels. From the large numbers of cancer cells that circulate in the blood stream, only < 0.01% of cells successfully deposit in distant tissues or organs. These few survive by covering themselves in platelets, thus disguising themselves and avoiding being recognised as a foreign object and being attacked by white blood cells.

Where do cancer cells spread to?

The precise mechanism of how a cancer cell moves to a distant site is not completely understood. Two theories have been proposed:

1. Anatomic spread – where cells move and settle in a organ/site not far from the primary site.
2. 'Seed and soil' theory – it is thought that some cells are drawn to specific organs.

The common places that cancer spreads to are the bone, lung, liver and brain. Some organs are ideal new homes for travelling cancer cells. For instance, the lungs have very thin capillaries with a single layer of endothelium and basement membrane, which is not much of a barrier for entry/exit of cancer cells, compared to arteries which

have an additional smooth muscle layer which may prevent spread. The liver is another easy target for metastatic disease as the hepatic portal vein breaks down into sinusoids which are not blood vessels, but are in direct contact with hepatocytes, making it easy for cancer cells to settle.

Some cancer cells spread more locally and extend directly into body cavities. For example, abdominal cancers such as colorectal and ovarian cancers often spread by cells dropping off or 'seeding' into the peritoneum.

What causes the DNA to become damaged?

As mentioned previously, some cancers cannot be attributed to any particular factor and may occur spontaneously. Although the exact causations of cancer are unknown, there is well-established evidence that some agents 'initiate' or 'promote' the development of cancer. These are known as *carcinogens*. Many are lifestyle-related factors, such as dietary, smoking or sun exposure, and are potentially preventable.

It is not a coincidence that 75% of cancers are *epithelial* (tissues that line the body inside and out) as these come in contact with environmental agents.

Age is a key risk factor in cancer. As we age, we are increasingly exposed to agents that cause damage to DNA and at the same time our immune system becomes less efficient and our repair genes become less effective.

It is important that causations of cancer are understood by the public so that people are able to appraise their own lifestyle behaviours and identify ways that they can change and reduce their likelihood of developing a cancer.

The following discussion presents current understanding of what are known to contribute to the development of cancer, split into three groups of

Reflection point

What are the causes of cancer that you might have read or heard about? Are these based on evidence you have read about or have you heard people you know talk about them? Where do people get their beliefs and attitudes from? What are these based on?

NMC Domain 1: 1.3
NMC Domain 3: 3.5

carcinogens: physical, biological and chemical factors.

Physical factors

Ionising radiation from natural and man-made sources is a known cause of cancer. As the radiation releases energy, the DNA sequence is altered, causing damage. This damage has been documented since its discovery in the 1800s, as well as in the aftermath of the nuclear bombings of Hiroshima and Nagasaki at the end of World War Two. The carcinogenic effect of radiation may be delayed for many years after exposure. In the past few years it has been reported that the use of therapeutic thoracic radiotherapy to treat Hodgkin's lymphoma in the 1970s has contributed to the development of breast cancer in the same group of patients 20 years later. X-rays use small amounts of radiation. Patients with long-term health needs may undergo multiple X-rays, therefore the use of all X-rays should be rationalised and restricted.

Ultraviolet radiation (UVA/UVB) from sun exposure has been clearly identified as causing 80% of *melanomas* and 90% of all *non-melanoma* (*basal cell* and *squamous cell carcinomas*) skin cancers. People with light eyes or hair who sunburn every easily are at more risk of developing skin cancer. The nature and length of exposure to the sun is significant. The higher intensity resulting in sunburn is more likely to result in melanoma (carrying a higher death rate). Squamous cell carcinoma is linked with chronic occupational sun exposure. The age at the time of exposure is also relevant; being sunburnt in childhood doubles the chances of developing melanoma. The use of sun beds remains extremely popular, especially with young adults, however this doubles the risk of *all* skin cancers.

Asbestos and exposure to coal dust has been unequivocally linked with *mesothelioma* (an aggressive type of lung cancer).

The physical and prolonged irritation of tissue such as in chronic wound/ulcers can damage the DNA and cause the development of *squamous cell carcinoma* around the edges of the wound.

Biological factors

Infections cause a number of cancers (approximately 10–20% worldwide). Although you cannot 'catch' cancer, certain viruses, bacteria and parasites can predispose individuals to develop cancer. Examples of such viruses are the following:

- Human papillomavirus (HPV) accounts for 80–90% of all cervical cancer cases as well as increasing numbers of oral cancers.
- Hepatitis B and C increase the risk of developing liver cancer by 80%.
- Epstein–Barr virus has been linked with Birkett's and Hodgkin's lymphoma.
- Human immunodeficiency virus (HIV) has been linked with Kaposi's sarcoma and non-Hodgkin's lymphoma.

Once in the body, some viruses have the ability to insert their own DNA into the human host, altering the sequence and subsequent protein production.

Parasites such as *Schistosoma haematobium* (common in India, Middle East and Africa) burrow into human skin, the pathogen then travels in the bloodstream and lodges in the bladder lining, increasing the risk of bladder cancer.

Bacteria such as *Helicobacter pylori* inhabit the stomachs of 50% of the world's population (although decreasing in Western countries). Eighty per cent of those infected with this Gram-negative bacteria will be asymptomatic, however it will cause inflammation of the stomach lining which may result in gastric cancer as well as ulcers.

Chemical factors

There are many chemical agents that have been linked to cancer, the most significant being tobacco – its consumption contributes to one-third of *all* cancers. Eighty-six per cent of all lung cancers are attributed to smoking, but cancer of the trachea, larynx, oral cavity, nasal cavity and sinuses, bladder, oesophagus, stomach, pancreas, cervix, kidney, liver, bowel and breast, as well as myeloid leukaemia, may all be linked to tobacco.

Smoking habits have altered across the world in the past 30 years, with a declining number of smokers in Western countries (especially men) and an increase in developing countries. In Western countries, there remains a socioeconomic divide – those less well off financially are more likely to smoke. With the increase in taxation, many smokers have started smoking 'roll ups'; these are more carcinogenic as there is little filtration. Others believe if they don't inhale fully that they are not at risk. In the UK there are growing numbers of teenage smokers with 15% of 15-year-olds smoking. The teenage years are significant in developing lifestyle habits, and smoking at this age establishes adult behaviours. As well as being influenced by the family, teenagers are influenced by their peers and advertising and become addicted in the same way as adults. It has been suggested that young smokers are at more risk of developing lung cancer, due to the high rate of cell growth during childhood.

Exposure to passive smoke has been clearly linked to lung cancer, increasing the risk by a quarter. A number of European countries (including the UK) and some states in the USA have banned smoking in public spaces (bars, restaurants, shops, etc.) to reduce passive inhalation of smoke.

As well as smoking tobacco, many individuals from South Asian and Native American cultures chew or keep the leaves of the tobacco plant between the lip and cheek. This practice is also linked to oral cancers.

Industrial processes and chemicals such as dioxins, benzene, vinyl chlorides, nickel and arsenic have all been connected with certain cancers and their use is subsequently restricted by environmental and health and safety regulations, such as the Control of Substances Hazardous to Health Regulations (COSHH) (Health and Safety Executive 2002) in the UK.

Diet is another important factor in the development of cancer. Approximately one-third of cancers are linked to dietary habits. However, this risk is incredibly difficult to quantify and specify as it is difficult to measure and identify what an individual's eating habits are over long periods of time and to isolate precise agents in food.

Salted and preserved foods have been linked with stomach cancer, however those who eat a diet of these foods may not eat a diet including plenty of fruit and vegetables. So it is difficult to say whether it is what is eaten or not eaten that is significant. An individual with colorectal cancer might have consumed a high-fat diet but at the same time ate little fruit and vegetables – is it the fat that contributed to the development of cancer or the lack of fruit and fibre?

It is proposed that some nutrients may protect cells from DNA damage, however it has been shown that if a particular nutritional element is extracted and taken as a 'supplement', this does not reduce the cancer in the same way as if the whole food was consumed. It is therefore important that a well-balanced nutritional diet is observed, with plenty of fruit and vegetables (of different colours – all having different micronutrients) and high in fibre.

Body weight, specifically obesity, has been linked with an increase risk of breast, bowel, uterine, oesophageal, pancreatic, kidney and gallbladder cancer. Diet is not the exclusive cause of obesity. Increased body weight is usually a result of overconsumption and lack of exercise, so physical activity is also relevant. As obesity continues to rise in Western countries, this presents significant health challenges to healthcare professionals in terms of cancer incidence as well as other conditions such as diabetes, heart disease, etc. An increased abdominal circumference (even if the body mass index (BMI) is within the normal range) has been suggested to increase the risk of cancer.

Sex hormones

The sex hormones (chemical messengers) produced in either the testes (androgens in men) or ovaries (oestrogen and progestin in women) influence cell division of their target cells: prostate, breast, ovary and uterus.

Diet influences the amount of hormone produced. For example, it has been suggested that men who consume a low-fat diet have reduced androgen (testosterone) levels and have a reduced risk of developing prostate cancer.

It has been well established that an increased amount of oestrogen, over a prolonged period of time, is linked to breast cancer (this is discussed shortly). Once a women reaches menopause, her ovaries stop producing oestrogen. However, the fatty tissue in the body continues to produce oestrogen – the more fatty tissue, the more oestrogen. Therefore, women who are overweight and have gone through the menopause have an increased amount of

oestrogen (than women with a normal BMI), increasing their risk of breast cancer.

In addition, the stages in a woman's reproductive history increase the likelihood of developing breast cancer due to the increased oestrogen produced and circulating:

- The age of menarche and menopause is significant – the younger a woman is when she starts her periods and the older she is when she finishes ovulating completely.
- Age at first full-term pregnancy.
- The number of live births.
- Length of time a woman breastfeeds.
- Exogenous hormones taken such as hormone replacement therapy (HRT).

Inherited damage

As highlighted previously, only 5–10% of cancers result from an inherited damaged gene. The most common inherited genetic defects are the tumour suppressor genes BRCA1 and BRCA2. These affect both men and women and carry an increased risk of developing breast cancer (50–80% lifetime risk). Ovarian cancer (20–60% lifetime risk) is associated with prostate, colorectal, and pancreatic cancer as well as ocular melanoma (cancer of the eye).

Other examples of inherited cancers are the following:

- Hereditary non-polyposis: this accounts for 5–10% of all colorectal cancers. Again, it is worth remembering that even if someone carries this defective gene they will not necessarily develop cancer, but they have a 25% chance of developing it by the age of 65 years old.
- Familial adenomatous polyposis (FAP): 1% of patients with colorectal cancer test positive for FAP. This, on the other hand, carries a 100% risk of developing cancer by the age of 50 years old. Both these conditions require regular surveillance by undergoing a sigmoidoscopy or colonoscopy.

- There are some hereditary syndromes associated with cancer, such as Li Frameni, Cowden and Von Hippel Lindau, however these are very rare. Usually, if a copy of a gene is inherited damaged from one parent, the second gene may be undamaged. This means the cell will behave normally. If the second copy becomes damaged then a cancer may develop. This is important to consider for health promotion. For instance, if an individual is found to carry a damaged BRCA gene then they may think 'it does not matter how I live my life, I will get cancer no matter what'. However, they are already genetically at risk of cancer so they could try to reduce their risk by following a healthy lifestyle and watching for any signs and symptoms.

Both men and women can be possible carriers of a faulty BRCA gene and either gender may develop cancer, however women are more likely to develop cancer. As a carrier, an individual will pass on the damaged gene on to any offspring. A detailed review of family history is essential to ascertain an individual's risk. Anyone who is worried about their family history can be referred to the genetic counselling team who will complete a family tree and assess the severity of risk. Those considered high risk will be offered additional surveillance and may consider prophylactic treatment. This is ethically challenging as there is a chance that they will not develop cancer. Although this knowledge may influence people to follow a healthy lifestyle and may make them more vigilant to detect early signs, it may have psychosocial implications and even an economic impact on health insurance and employment.

 Activity

Choose one of the common cancers you have heard about (it might be cancer that is very common in your local community). Find out what the incidence and mortality rates are and what the possible agents are that may contribute to the development of this cancer. What simple health promotion strategies could help reduce the cancer risk?

NMC Domain 1: 1.3
NMC Domain 2: 2.6
NMC Domain 3: 3.5

References

Health and Safety Executive, 2002. The Control of Substances Hazardous to Health regulations. Approved code of practice and guidance, 5th ed. HSE, London. Online. Available at: http://www.hse.gov.uk/coshh/ (accessed May 2011).

Waugh, A., Grant, A., 2010. Ross and Wilson anatomy and physiology in health and illness. Churchill Livingstone, Edinburgh.

Further reading

Kearney, N., Richardson, A., 2006. Nursing patients with cancer: principles and practice. Churchill Livingstone, Edinburgh.

King, R.J.B., Robins, M.W., 2006. Cancer biology, 3rd ed. Prentice Hall, Harlow.

Pecorino, L., 2008. Molecular biology of cancer: mechanisms, targets and therapeutics, 2nd ed. Oxford University Press, Oxford.

Scotting, P., 2010. Cancer: a beginners guide. Oneworld, Oxford.

3 How the cancer situation can be improved

CHAPTER AIMS

- To understand how to prevent cancer developing
- To identify how survival rates can be improved
- To explore public health approaches to detecting cancer at an earlier stage

How to prevent cancer developing

Having identified the possible causations of cancer, we have an opportunity to use this knowledge to inform and influence individual lifestyles and behaviours. This can be done on several levels:

- Government and local policy: for example, the banning of smoking in public places; taxation of cigarettes and alcohol; national vaccination programmes, such as the human papillomavirus vaccine for teenage girls (16 and 18 strains); health and safety at work: Control of substances hazardous to health (COSHH) regulations and advertising (COSHH 2002).
- Individually: everyone has the opportunity to make small changes in their lifestyle to reduce their cancer risk, such as giving up smoking; eating a well-balanced diet with plenty of fruit and vegetables; safe sexual practice (using a condom); applying sun screen appropriately (correct sun protection factor (SPF) for skin type and sun intensity, applied at correct time intervals); and taking exercise to maintain a healthy body mass index.

As healthcare professionals, we have a responsibility to promote and provide information to assist individuals to make healthy lifestyle choices, even if this is in a very small way. Many nurses working in acute care environments consider that their role is to care for 'sick' people and do not recognise the opportunities to improve the health of their patients and/or families. This needn't be heavy handed – it might be during a routine admission or assessment. We often ask patients whether they smoke, but what do we do with this information? This is a good opportunity to gently enquire whether the individual has considered or has even tried to give up smoking. If they show interest we should either refer or signpost them to the local smoking cessation programme or provide information on the national telephone helpline/Website. We don't need to have all the answers. It is about providing the information to direct people to existing services that can support them. If they are not interested in changing their behaviours, they will soon tell us. It is their choice how they live their lives and we have no right to judge them.

Reflection point

Reflect back on previous placements/ experiences. What health promotion opportunities were there and what could you have done differently?

NMC Domain 1: 1.3; 1.8
NMC Domain 2: 2.6
NMC Domain 3: 3.5
NMC Domain 4: 4.1

How survival rates can be improved

As well as preventing cancers in the first place, detecting cancers early in their development also reduces the risk of death. The majority of cancers are identified by individuals after they notice a change in their body appearance or function. When the sign or symptom has become noticeable, they seek medical advice. Unfortunately by this point the cancer has often become sizable and may have spread, making it difficult to treat, and the overall outcome may be less successful.

Activity

Talk to a patient with cancer (who is happy to share their story). Find out about the initial signs and symptoms they experienced prior to diagnosis. Alternatively, listen to a patient's story on the healthtalkonline.org Website, for example: http://www.healthtalkonline .org/Cancer/Colorectal_Cancer/Topic/ 1061/ (accessed November 2011)

NMC Domain 1: 1.4
NMC Domain 2: 2.3
NMC Domain 3: 3.2; 3.5; 3.7

Early detection of cancer depends on people knowing what to look for and seeking prompt advice from their doctor (Box 3.1). Education is essential for people to understand how the body works; knowing what is normal for our own bodies helps us detect when something changes. Fear can play a large part in delaying seeking help and is often driven by 'I don't want to know' or 'they won't be able to do anything for me'. These feelings may be based on previous family experiences or out-of-date

Box 3.1 Signs of cancer for men and women

- An unusual lump or swelling anywhere on the body
- A change in the size, shape or colour of a mole
- A sore that won't heal after several weeks
- An unexplained pain or ache that lasts longer than 4 weeks
- A cough or croaky voice that lasts longer than 3 weeks
- Unexplained weight loss or heavy night sweats
- An unusual breast change
- Persistent difficulty swallowing or indigestion
- Problems passing urine
- Blood in urine
- Blood in bowel motions
- A change to more frequent bowel motions that lasts longer than 6 weeks
- A mouth or tongue ulcer that lasts longer than 3 weeks
- Bleeding from the vagina after the menopause or between periods

information. It is important to educate people that cancer can often be treated and have a good outcome if it is detected and treated early, emphasising that it is vitally important to note any changes in body function or appearance.

 Activity

Identify simple ways you raise the awareness of the signs and symptoms of cancer in the individuals you meet.

NMC Domain 1: 1.3; 1.4
NMC Domain 2: 2.6
NMC Domain 3: 3.5; 3.7; 3.8
NMC Domain 4: 4.1

Screening

A possible way of detecting a cancer *before* symptoms develop is through screening. The primary aim of screening is to identify a cancer at an early stage, so that treatment can be prompt and the impact of treatment may be minimised and more successful, although this is not always the case. The general population are targeted for screening, although programmes select specific age groups or high-risk individuals.

Wilson and Junger (1968) developed 10 principles (for the World Health Organisation) that should govern a national screening programme:

1. The condition should be an important health issue.
2. The natural history of the disease should be well understood.
3. There should be a recognisable early stage which is responsive to treatment.
4. A suitable and acceptable test should exist.
5. The population to be screened can be identified.
6. An interval period must be decided upon.
7. There needs to be adequate facilities to cope with the abnormalities detected.

8. Treatment must be available and acceptable to the population.
9. The cost of screening must be viable.
10. Overall the benefits of screening should outweigh the harm.

 Reflection point

Consider Wilson and Junger's (1968) (see References) 10 principles of screening. Why do we have a breast screening programme and not a prostate screening programme?

NMC Domain 1: 1.4
NMC Domain 2: 2.6
NMC Domain 3: 3.5

Cervical screening

Cervical screening is fairly unique in the fact that it does not just detect cancer at an earlier stage but it can prevent cancer developing. This is because there is a recognised pre-cancerous stage called *carcinoma in situ* (CIN). If untreated, this condition will almost definitely develop into a cancer. However, if this is detected during screening then the affected tissues can be removed and the individual does not develop cancer. It is estimated that screening, the detection of CIN and prompt treatment can prevent 75% of cervical cancers.

The programme screens women between the ages of 25 to 49 every 3 years and 50 to 64 every 5 years. Women over 65 years who have not been screened since age 50 or have had an abnormal result can request screening. In 2005, the method of screening was changed to liquid-based cytology (involves brushing the cervix and suspending the brush in a medium before it is reviewed) to increase the reliability of the test.

The evidence in favour of screening for cancer of the cervix is convincing. Of the

4 million women in the UK invited for screening in 2007–2008, 3.3 million were tested and 93% were negative (NHS Cervical Screening Programme Statistical Bulletin (England 2009–10)).

Although commenced in the mid 1960s, the number of women attending cervical cancer screening has been sporadic and the number has declined slightly in the past 10 years. Of those women invited for screening, 78.9% attended. Women in the younger age groups have declined more rapidly.

Breast screening

The UK NHS Breast Screening Programme (1986) was the first of its kind in the world and national coverage was achieved by the mid 1990s. There have been numerous adjustments to the programme since this time. Currently all women aged 47 to 73 years are sent a letter inviting them to attend for a mammography every 3 years. Women over 73 can request screening.

In 2007–2008, of the 2.5 million women invited for screening, a total of 2 million were screened and 16 449 cancers were detected (Cancer Research UK 2010). Breast screening is well established and shown to be effective, lowering mortality rates (55–69 years) and saving approximately 1250 lives per year.

Colorectal screening

Colorectal cancer is often diagnosed very late, when the cancer has become inoperable and may have spread. This is because there are very few early signs or symptoms due to the amount of space in the abdomen. For this reason, the early detection of colorectal cancer through screening is very attractive. Colorectal cancer screening was introduced in the UK in 2008 for 60–69-year-olds and is due to be extended to 70–79-year-olds in the near future. Individuals receive a

screening kit in the post asking them to provide a small sample of faeces which is then returned in the post to investigate the presence of faecal occult blood (FOB). In the event of a positive result, the individual will be recalled for a colonoscopy.

The bowel screening pilot study suggests that death rates can be reduced by 15–20% and it is estimated that by 2025 the screening programme could save more than 2000 lives every year. The use of flexible sigmoidoscopy as a screening tool has been shown in trials to be promising and may be introduced in the future.

Overall, it is often challenging to get people to attend screening, due to a lack of understanding of the programme or the test itself, logistical difficulties such as transport, child care, getting time of work, etc., or the fear of diagnosis (ignorance is bliss).

Although most people attending understand that screening involves a test to identify physical changes that *might* be a result of cancer, they also attend so they can feel reassured that they do not have cancer. If they are recalled for further investigation, it may be a complete surprise as they may not have any signs or symptoms.

No test is perfect and all screening methods will result in a number of 'false negatives'. This is where an individual is told they are all clear but in fact they do have a cancer that has not been detected. Conversely, there are a number of false positives, where individuals are recalled for further investigation but do not have cancer. This can be psychologically distressing before the true results are reported.

There is a common misconception that screening is a diagnostic tool, but an individual cannot be diagnosed without a number of additional investigations, in particular a pathological sample.

References

Cancer Research UK, 2010. Breast screening statistics. Online. Available at: http://info.cancerresearchuk.org/ cancerstats/types/breast/screening/ (accessed November 2011).

Health and Safety Executive, 2002. Control of substances hazardous to health (COSHH). HSE. London.

NHS Breast Screening Programme, 1986. The Forrest report. Online. Available at: http://www.cancerscreening.nhs.uk/ breastscreen/publications/ forrest-report.html (accessed November 2011).

NHS Cervical Screening Programme Statistical Bulletin (England 2009–10). Online. Available at: www.cancerscreening.nhs.uk (accessed May 2011).

Wilson, J.M.G., Junger, G., 1968. Principles and practice of screening for disease. Public Health Paper 34. World Health Organisation, Geneva.

Further reading

Corner, J., Bailey, C. (Eds.), 2008. Cancer nursing: care in context, 2nd ed. Blackwell, Oxford.

Websites

NHS Cancer Screening Programmes Website for England, http://www.cancerscreening .nhs.uk/index.html (accessed May 2011).

UK Screening Portal, http://www.screening .nhs.uk/ (accessed May 2011).

Healthtalkonline, http://www.healthtalkonline. org/Cancer/ (accessed May 2011).

4

How cancer is diagnosed and the impact of diagnosis

CHAPTER AIMS

- To understand how cancer is investigated
- To understand how cancers are classified and staged
- To appreciate the impact of a cancer diagnosis

How cancer is investigated

Whether an individual is asymptomatic and the cancer is detected during a routine screening programme or at another health event (such as a routine preoperative chest X-ray) or whether they present with significant signs and symptoms, most patients will be referred to an appropriate clinician/consultant. At this point, the most likely causes of the sign/symptom is considered and further investigations are undertaken to make a definitive diagnosis. There are a whole range of tests that are done, depending on the suspected site, but generally patients undergo one or a few of the following:

- Positron emission tomography (PET).
- Computed tomography (CT).
- Bone scan.
- Magnetic resonance imaging (MRI).
- X-ray.
- Tumour markers as well as other blood tests.

Tumour markers are hormones, antigens or enzymes produced by the cancer itself or by tissues stimulated by the cancer. However, the presence of a tumour marker does not always mean a patient has cancer. For instance, a raised prostate-specific antigen (PSA) may indicate prostate cancer. However, an individual may have an increased PSA due to a benign prostate condition or physical stimulation of the prostate such as sexual intercourse. Other common tumour markers are CA-125 for ovarian and colorectal gastric cancer, and carcinoembryonic antigen (CEA) for breast, colorectal and lung cancer. Immunohistochemistry (IHC) is used to test whether a patient is over expressing these receptors. For example, 30–40% of patients with breast cancer are positive for human epidermal receptors (HER2). If positive, the type of cancer may be more aggressive but the patient may be a good candidate for the drug Herceptin (trastuzumab).

Depending on the type of cancer, some patients may have a test to see if hormones are affecting the growth of the cancer, such as prostate and breast cancer. A significant number of breast cancers have increased *oestrogen* growth receptors on the cell surface; this means that the cancer grows more easily in the presence of oestrogen. These cancers are known as hormone sensitive or hormone positive (ER+). Other breast cancers may be *progesterone* sensitive (PR+). If a breast cancer is not sensitive to oestrogen, progesterone or HER2 then it is *triple negative.* Triple negative breast cancers tend to be more aggressive and develop in younger women.

A cancer diagnosis can only be made when a sample of tissue has been taken, usually in the form of a *biopsy* (tissue) or *cytology* (body fluids). When these have been analysed, the *histopathology* (type of cancer) can be identified and classified.

To identify if the cancer has spread to any of the local lymph nodes, sometimes a *sentinel node biopsy* is performed. This involves injecting a blue dye (and sometimes a radioactive liquid) into areas close to the cancer, while the patient undergoes surgical removal of the lump. The lymph nodes are then scanned or observed to see which lymph node(s) take up the dye/radioactive liquid. The node that shows up is known as the sentinel node and is removed and sent to be tested for cancer. This helps the staging process and may aid treatment decisions, which may mean less treatment and less long-term side effects.

By the time investigations are underway, the majority of patients will be informed of the possible causes of the symptoms, and by the time the results are confirmed, the news of cancer is not a complete surprise. Most patients are informed of the diagnosis in the outpatient setting or on a general medical or surgical ward, so you may not witness diagnosis being given on an oncology placement.

 Activity

The Royal College of Radiologists has produced a range of patient information on interventional radiology, diagnostic radiology and oncology procedures. Visit the following Website and look up some of the investigations you have heard about on placement or have witnessed:

http://www.rcr.ac.uk/content.aspx?PageID=323 (accessed May 2011).

NMC Domain 3: 3.1; 3.2; 3.3; 3.6

 Activity

Watch a biopsy being performed. Write a brief reflection on the procedure. Think about preparing the patient and maintaining safety and patient comfort. Find out how the specimen is processed.

NMC Domain 1: 1.4
NMC Domain 2: 2.4
NMC Domain 3: 3.1; 3.2; 3.6

 Activity

Visit or escort a patient to the radiology department and observe a scan. Alternatively, visit the Macmillan Website:

http://www.macmillan.org.uk/Cancerinformation/Cancerinformation.aspx (accessed May 2011).

On this Website, look at one type of cancer and identify the common investigations that a patient may undergo. For example, lung cancer investigations can be found at:

http://www.macmillan.org.uk/Cancerinformation/Cancertypes/Lung/Symptomsdiagnosis/Diagnosistests/Tests.aspx (accessed May 2011).

NMC Domain 3: 3.1; 3.3; 3.6

How cancers are classified and staged

Once a diagnosis has been established, a referral to an appropriate surgeon or oncologist (cancer specialist) is made to review the situation, stage and classify the cancer in order for treatment to be planned.

From a psychological perspective, the point of diagnosis is usually not the start of the story for the patient; they may have experienced symptoms for some months. Receiving a definitive diagnosis may be a relief, providing answers to questions and confirming what is wrong, and it may remove the anxiety associated with the sense of uncertainty. For others it may be a total shock.

 Activity

Identify a patient with cancer. Look through their medical notes to find out which investigations they had in order to reach a diagnosis (CT, MRI, PET, biopsy, bone scan, etc.).

NMC Domain 3: 3.2; 3.3

Classification

The results from the investigations may help to establish the type, position, size, grade and stage of the cancer. These will all be used to ensure an appropriate treatment is selected, along with a thorough assessment of the patient (this is discussed in Ch. 5). It is very important that the right words are used to describe all aspects of the cancer so that healthcare professionals are aware of the situation and the patient is not confused with too many different medical terms.

The word *tumour* is often used and, although it means 'lump', it is an ambiguous term and can mean either *benign* or *malignant*. This can confuse patients. If they are told they have a tumour, they may assume that they have a benign condition, when they actually have a malignant cancer. Although benign tumours can cause problems due to their size; be painful or unsightly; press on other body organs; take up space inside the skull (for example, like a brain tumour); and release hormones that affect how the body works, they are *not* cancers. Cancers are made up of malignant cells which are discussed in Chapter 2, so it is best to avoid the use of the word 'tumour', and use the word 'cancer' so that patients do not become confused. The main differences between benign and malignant tumours are given in Table 4.1.

Table 4.1 Difference between benign and malignant tumours

Benign	Malignant
Slow growing	Usually faster growing
Encapsulated	Irregular in shape
Cells appear normal under the microscope	Spreads locally and destroys the surrounding tissues
Does not spread to other parts of the body	Spreads to other parts of the body

In the clinical setting, tumours are described according to their *histogenesis* (the names are specific to the cells/tissues from which they arise) and are often named from Greek and Latin terms. In general, benign tumours end in the suffix '-oma' which means 'lump' in Latin. Malignant cancers usually have a prefix to the '-oma' which is related to the tissue of origin. For example, malignant tumours that derive from epithelial tissues (lining tissues) are called *carcinomas*. Carcinomas account for 75% of all cancers and there are two types of carcinoma – *adenocarcinoma* (cancer in glandular tissue) and *squamous cell carcinoma* (cancer in squamous epithelium). Cancers arising in the connective tissues (bone, cartilage, muscle, fibrous tissue) are called *sarcomas* (accounting for 20% of cancers) and cancers in the neural tissue are called *blastomas*.

The specific names of tumours (both benign and malignant) are also made up of the specific tissue in the body (Table 4.2). So a benign, non-malignant tumour in the unstriated smooth muscle would be called a 'leio-my-oma' and a malignant cancerous tumour in the unstriated smooth muscle would be a 'leio-myo-sarc-oma'. There are

some exceptions to this rule. For instance, using the rules above, melanoma and lymphoma sound like they are benign tumours when in fact they are malignant.

Other cancers are named after the researcher who first described them, for example Hodgkin's lymphoma and Kaposi's sarcoma.

Staging

To ascertain the extent that the cancer has grown, many cancers are staged using the *TNM classification* (Sobin et al 2010). This divides cancers into groups to provide a precise description:

- Tumour (T): identifies the primary tumour, size and infiltration.
- Node (N): identifies lymph node involvement.
- Metastatic (M): represents presence or absence of distant metastases.

Staging is important to indicate prognosis (likely outcome) as well as guide decisions regarding treatment. For instance, if a cancer is very large or if it has spread to a distant part then surgery will not remove the cancer completely, and an alternative treatment will be considered. Staging also aids communication between healthcare professionals and to measure the success of treatment.

There are other methods of staging cancers. For example, Table 4.3 outlines Dukes staging of colorectal cancer (Dukes 1932).

Table 4.2 Naming of tumours

Adeno-	Glandular tissue
Haemo-	Blood
Angio-	Vessels
Lipo-	Fat
Osteo-	Bone
Myo-	Muscle
Rhabdo-	Striated muscle
Leio-	Unstriated (smooth) muscle
Chondro-	Cartilage
Endo-	Lining

Table 4.3 Dukes staging of colorectal cancer

Stage	Tumour	Nodes	Metastatic spread
Dukes A	T1	N0	M0
Dukes B1	T3	N0	M0
Dukes B2	T4	N0	M0
Dukes C1	T1 or T2	N1 or N2	M0
Dukes C2	T3 or T4	N1 or N2	M0
Dukes D	Any size tumour	Any number of nodes	M1 distant metastases

Grading

Grading refers to how mutated the cells have become. The more a cell mutates, the more it may lose all resemblance to the normal tissue from which it arises. Grading is based on the appearance of the cancer under the microscope. Sometimes it is impossible to tell what type of cell a mutated cell was originally, and this leads to the diagnosis of *unknown primary*. The extent to which a cancer resembles the normal tissue is known as the degree of *differentiation* (Table 4.4).

The differentiation or grade provides some indication of how mutated the cells look and how similar they are in terms of function compared to the normal cells. This is clinically helpful to predict prognosis. For example, when staging breast cancer, the *Nottingham Prognostic Index* (NPI) is often used (Haybrittle, Blamey and Elston 1982). This is a formula which gives an indication of how successful treatment might be, by considering the size of the cancer, whether or not the cancer has spread to the lymph nodes under the arm (and, if so, how many nodes are affected) and the grade of the cancer.

Table 4.4 Grading of cancer

Well differentiated	Grade I Resembles normal cell – low grade
Moderately differentiated	Grade II Some similarities to normal cell
Poorly differentiated	Grade III Very immature, little resemblance to normal cell
Undifferentiated (anaplastic/ dedifferentiated)	Grade IV No resemblance to original tissue – high grade

The formula is: NPI = (0.2 × cancer diameter in cm) + lymph node stage + cancer grade.

The lymph node stage is rated 1 if there are no nodes affected; 2 if up to three glands are affected or 3 if more than three glands are affected.

The cancer grade is scored 1 for a grade I less aggressive appearance, 2 if a grade II intermediate appearance or 3 for a grade III, more aggressive appearance.

Applying the formula gives scores which fall into three bands:

1. Less than 3.4 suggests a good outcome with a high chance of a cure.
2. 3.4–5.4 suggests an intermediate level with a moderate chance of a cure.
3. More than 5.4 suggests a worse outlook with less chance of a cure.

Activity

Select a patient you are caring for, either an individual who is in hospital or one being cared for in the community. Look through their medical notes to identify what the name of their cancer is, how this relates to the type of tissue the cancer is present in and what the staging and grade of the cancer are. Discuss with your mentor how this information has influenced the patient's treatment and nursing care.

NMC Domain 3: 3.1; 3.2

The staging and grading information will be discussed at a multiprofessional meeting where all possible treatment options will be identified. All the possible options will be explained to the patient to help them decide which treatment to undergo. Chapter 8 outlines different treatment options and explores why one treatment might be chosen over another.

The impact of a cancer diagnosis

It may seem odd, but you may not have the opportunity to witness someone being told they have cancer while you are on your cancer/palliative placement. This is because individuals are often admitted to a medical or surgical ward with signs and symptoms which, once investigated, are found to result from cancer. From this point, the patient will be referred to an appropriate specialist who will pursue further tests. It is important that the person delivering the news is prepared; they should have as much information as they can and have undergone training in breaking significant news.

The East Midlands Cancer Network (2010) outlines 'eleven well recognised steps to breaking bad news' in their nationally recognised guidelines (Box 4.1)

These steps provide healthcare professionals (of all grades) with practical help in all care settings, to communicate bad news in an effective manner. These guidelines can be looked at shortly before seeing a patient, but are not intended to be used rigidly as everyone reacts differently to being given the news they have cancer. Predicting how someone might react is equally as difficult as it is to predict what the impact of diagnosis or outcome might be. Reaction is often influenced by whether the individual was expecting the news. If the cancer is identified during a routine screening and they don't have any symptoms, then it might be a complete shock. For others who have experienced symptoms over a long period of time, it might be a relief to have an answer to the cause

Box 4.1 The East Midlands Cancer Network (2010) guidelines for communicating bad news with patients and their families

- Step one – preparation and scene setting
- Step two – what does the patient know?
- Step three – is more information wanted at that time?
- Step four – give a warning shot
- Step five – allow patient to decline information at this time
- Step six – explain (if requested)
- Step seven – elicit and listen to concerns
- Step eight – encourage ventilation of feeling
- Step nine – summary and plan
- Step ten – offer availability and support
- Step eleven – communicate with the team

of the problems, often enabling the symptoms to be alleviated by treatment.

Previous experience and knowledge of cancer may influence how individuals comprehend their situation. An individual who has observed or cared for friends and family with a cancer may use this experience to foresee what their experience is likely to be and what they expect to happen. These encounters also affect an individual's attitudes and beliefs regarding what caused the cancer and what the likely outcome might be. One of the difficulties is that no two cancer experiences can be compared, even if they are cancers of the same anatomical site. Despite this, patients will often compare experiences with other patients or people they know who have had cancer, even if is a completely different type of cancer, having completely different treatment, with a completely different outcome. Previous experiences may also influence a patient when they are deciding on treatment options.

The stage and grade of cancer may or may not affect the impact, so someone who is diagnosed with an advanced, aggressive, metastatic cancer may not necessarily be more distressed than someone who is diagnosed with a small, non-aggressive local cancer.

The way a diagnosis is given and who gives the news can influence the situation. It is normally a consultant who imparts the news initially, but the role of the nurse is important, allowing the patient and family time to digest the information to clarify what has been said and to answer questions.

⟨✦⟩ Reflection point

What else might affect someone's reaction to a cancer diagnosis? How might an individual react? What sort of emotions might they experience?

Visit The Patient Experience Website to watch a video of a patient's experience of diagnosis and the patient pathway:

http://www.patient-experience.com/index.php/diagnosis-of-breast-cancer-blog/ (accessed November 2011).

NMC Domain 1: 2.4
NMC Domain 3: 3.4; 3.9

One of the most common questions patients want to know is 'Why me?' and 'What have I done?' It is a normal reaction to try and find meaning in a situation and identify the reason something has happened. However, these questions are impossible to answer and may cause enormous angst. A diagnosis can be seen as a punishment or they may feel guilty for their life choices or behaviours (especially if they perceive their actions may have contributed to the cancer developing). People might want to blame something or somebody, often themselves, asking questions such as 'Why did I smoke when I knew it was bad for me?' or 'Why didn't I go to the doctor earlier?' Other reactions might be disbelief – 'How could this have happened?' Denial is a common reaction – 'They have made a mistake with the results. . .' – or using distraction by focusing on other things to ignore the trauma of the immediate situation. Some may not want to talk about the cancer or may not wish to say the word 'cancer'. Some patients are angry, often at the perceived (or actual) inadequacies of the health service.

At the point of diagnosis, there is an enormous sense of uncertainty, associated with many questions:

- Can it be treated?
- What treatments are there?
- Am I going to die?
- How long have I got?

It may take a number of weeks and months before some of these questions can be answered (some may never have an answer) and, during this time, patients require information to help them deal with the many unanswered questions. To help them cope with the uncertainty, some patients may rekindle a religious faith while others may lose faith in religion. Either way, it is vital that a therapeutic relationship is developed between the patient and healthcare team, so that the patient feels that the healthcare team are knowledgeable, experienced and will do the very best they can.

On the healthtalkonline Website, you can listen to patients' experiences and what it feels like to be diagnosed with cancer: http://www.healthtalkonline.org/Cancer/ (accessed November 2011).

 Reflection point

> What questions do you think a newly diagnosed individual might ask?
> How can you prepare for these questions?
>
> NMC Domain 2: 2.2; 2.3; 2.4
> NMC Domain 3: 3.8

 Activity

> Read Thain and Palmer (2010) (see References) to explore some of the techniques and strategies to minimise shock and distress (for example 'the SPIKES protocol).
>
> NMC Domain 1: 1.9
> NMC Domain 2: 2.1; 2.2; 2.3; 2.4; 2.5
> NMC Domain 4: 4.2

Once diagnosis has been given, patients need time and support to try to comprehend what is happening to them, so they can adjust to their situation. This is generally a difficult time for all who know the person (in varying degrees). Friends, colleagues, neighbours and family may avoid seeing the individual as they don't know what to say and worry they will say the wrong thing. This may result in the individual feeling isolated and stigmatised.

 Activity

> List what might be the implications of a diagnosis of cancer on an individual:
> - physically
> - emotionally
> - socially
> - economically
>
> NMC Domain 3: 3.3; 3.4; 3.7

It is vital that the individual knows who they can contact and talk to regarding their anxieties and questions. Many clinical areas use an assessment tool such as the 'distress thermometer' (Fig. 4.1) to help patients and healthcare professionals identify specific issues patients might be experiencing. Assessment tools like this one are quick and easy to use, allowing the patient to identify any problems (physical, social, economic or psychological) they may be experiencing. Once patients and healthcare professionals have recognised the patients' problems, then something can be done to support them. This doesn't mean to say healthcare professionals have 'all the answers' as often there are not any definitive answers and we can't always 'solve the situation'. Often it is enough to sit with the patient and family and listen to their concerns: some situations may require the healthcare professional to provide information; other situations may require the healthcare professional to offer direct help; still other situations may require a referral to other health professionals or other agencies (support groups/charities) for specialised intervention/care/support. This type of assessment and intervention is covered in Section 2 where aspects of a cancer patient's experience are explored.

First please circle the number (0-10) that best describes how much distress in general you have been experiencing over the past week, including today.

Second, if any of the following has been a problem for you over the past week, including today, please tick the box next to it. Leave it blank if it does not apply to you. Then rank your top 4 difficulties (1 would be the biggest problem, 4 would be your fourth biggest concern).

THERMOMETER

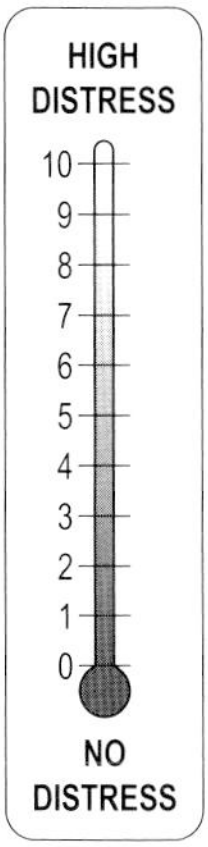

HIGH DISTRESS
10
9
8
7
6
5
4
3
2
1
0
NO DISTRESS

RANKING

Practical Problems
☐ Child care
☐ Housing
☐ Finances
☐ Transportation
☐ Work/school

Family Problems
☐ Dealing with children
☐ Dealing with partner

Emotional Problems
☐ Depression
☐ Fears
☐ Nervousness
☐ Sadness
☐ Worry
☐ Anger
☐ Unable to make plans

Spiritual/religious concerns
☐ Loss of faith
☐ Relating to God
☐ Loss of meaning or purpose of life

Other problems ....

RANKING

Physical Problems
☐ Appearance
☐ Bathing/dressing
☐ Breathing
☐ Changes in urination
☐ Constipation
☐ Diarrhoea
☐ Eating
☐ Fatigue/Tiredness
☐ Feeling swollen
☐ Fevers
☐ Getting around
☐ Indigestion
☐ Mouth sores
☐ Nausea
☐ Nose dry/congested
☐ Pain
☐ Sexual
☐ Skin dry/itchy
☐ Sleep
☐ Tingling in hands/feet
☐ Metallic taste in mouth

Patient details	Signed by staff member:	Today's date:
		DURATION OF INTERVIEW: (in minutes)
	Diagnosis:	

Highest ranked concerns	RATING	Description and history of problem	Plan of action
1.			
2.			
3.			
4.			

Fig 4.1 The distress thermometer (adapted from Roth et al (1998) and National Comprehensive Cancer Network NCCN (2007))

References

Dukes, C.E., 1932. The classification of cancer of the rectum. Journal of pathological bacteriology 35, 323.

East Midlands Cancer Network, 2010. The guidelines for communicating bad news with patients and their families: significant news. Online. Available at: http://www .eastmidlandscancernetwork.nhs.uk/ Library/BreakingBadNewsGuidelines.pdf (accessed May 2011).

Haybrittle, J.L., Blamey, R.W., Elston, C.W., 1982. A prognostic index in primary breast cancer. British Journal of cancer 45 (3), 361–366.

National Comprehensive Cancer Network, 2007. Clinical practice guidelines in oncology: distress management. Online. Available at: http://www.nccn.org/ professionals/physician_gls/f_guidelines .asp (accessed November 2011).

Roth, A.J., Kornblith, A.B., Batel-Copel, L., et al., 1998. Rapid screening for psychologic distress in men with prostate carcinoma: a pilot study. Cancer 82, 1904–1908.

Sobin, L.H., Gospodarowicz, M.K., Wittekind, C.H. (Eds.), 2010. TNM classification of malignant tumours. 7th ed. Wiley–Liss, New York.

Thain, C., Palmer, C., 2010. Strategies to ensure effective and empathetic delivery of bad news. Cancer Nursing Practice 9 (9), 24–27.

Further reading

Bultz, B.C., Carlson, L.E., 2005. Emotional distress: the sixth vital sign in cancer care. J. Clin. Oncol. 23 (26), 6440–6441.

Campbell, J., 2007. Understanding social support for patients with cancer. Nurs. Times 103 (23), 28–29.

Edwards, B., Clarke, V., 2004. The psychological impact of a cancer diagnosis on families: the influence of family functioning and patients' illness characteristics on depression and anxiety. Psychooncology 13 (8), 562–576.

Pitceathly, C., Maguire, P., 2004. The psychological impact of cancer on patients' partners and other key relatives: a review. Eur. J. Cancer 39 (11), 1517–1524.

Ryan, H., Schofield, P., Cockburn, J., et al., 2005. How to recognize and manage psychological distress in cancer patients. Eur. J. Cancer Care (Engl.) 14, 7–15.

Saaegrov, S., Haling, A., 2004. What is it like living with a diagnosis of cancer? Eur. J. Cancer Care (Engl.) 13, 145–153.

Stringer, S., 2008. Psychosocial impact of cancer. Cancer Nursing Practice 7 (7), 32–34, 37.

Websites

Macmillan patient information, http://www .macmillan.org.uk/Home.aspx (accessed May 2011).

Royal College of Radiologists patient information, http://www.rcr.ac.uk/ content.aspx?PageID=323 (accessed May 2011).

The Patient Experience Website, http://www .patient-experience.com/index.php/ diagnosis-of-breast-cancer-blog/ (accessed July 2011).

5 Principles of palliative care nursing

CHAPTER AIMS

- To explore the historical developments of palliative care
- To explain the meaning of palliative care
- To understand the core terms used within palliative care
- To understand palliative care today
- To explore the ethical debates in palliative care

The historical developments of palliative care

The core role of palliative care is about relieving symptoms in advanced disease while supporting both patients and relatives by providing holistic-focused care.

The term 'palliative care' emerged with the growth of the hospice movement in England in the 1960s yet has its roots back to fifteenth century international history. The words 'palliate' and 'pallium' are both from late Latin, meaning to 'cloak or conceal'. The aim of palliative care is to cloak and conceal the symptoms of the disease rather than provide a cure. For example, a patient with a brain tumour might be experiencing confusion, nausea and pain due to inflammation of the cerebral meninges in the brain due to growth and pressure from the cancer. Administering a steroid like dexamethasone may help to reduce this inflammation and settle these distressing symptoms. This treatment, while helping to attain comfort, will not stop the tumour growth. However, symptoms are hopefully 'cloaked and concealed' and comfort is achieved for the patient with the overall aim of increasing the quality of life.

Growth of the hospice movement

As far back as 2000 years ago, institutions across the world have cared for weary travellers. These included the homeless, pregnant women and migrant workers who were offered food, warmth and shelter. Often the ill and vulnerable would remain at these places of refuge to be cared for until they died. The term 'hospice care' emerged from these places of care: 'hospes' is Latin for host; 'hospitium' is Latin for hospitality. The term 'hospice' was first applied to the care of the dying by Madame Jeanne Garnier who founded the Dames de Calaire hospice in Lyon, France in 1842.

Activity

Find out where the nearest hospice is to where you are studying. What is the history of this hospice? Find out about the types of patients who are cared for there. Patients on your practice placement might be aware of this hospice, it might be something they need explaining about or are fearful of. They may have a family member or friend who has died there. Having the information to give is important in helping to reduce anxiety. The hospice may be a place you can visit from your 'hub' practice placement. Some of you may even have your main placement in a hospice.

NMC Domain 1: 1.1; 1.4; 1.6
NMC Domain 2: 2.1; 2.4; 2.5
NMC Domain 3: 3.9
NMC Domain 4: 4.1

The meaning of palliative care

The World Health Organisation (WHO) defines palliative care as an approach that improves the quality of life of patients and their families facing the problems associated with life-threatening illness, through the prevention and relief of suffering by means of early identification and impeccable assessment and treatment of pain and other problems, physical, psychosocial and spiritual. Palliative care:

- provides relief from pain and other distressing symptoms
- affirms life and regards dying as a normal process
- intends neither to hasten nor postpone death

- integrates the psychological and spiritual aspects of patient care
- offers a support system to help patients live as actively as possible until death
- offers a support system to help the family cope during the patient's illness and in their own bereavement
- uses a team approach to address the needs of patients and their families, including bereavement counselling if indicated
- will enhance quality of life, and may also positively influence the course of illness (WHO 2003).

This chapter now considers each of the eight parts of the WHO definition of palliative care and gives you a short activity for each to help you think about nursing actions that can ensure the definition is achieved in any practice area.

Provides relief from pain and other distressing symptoms

Often the focus of care can be on relieving a physical pain without considering wider issues for the patient. Dame Cicely Saunders, the doctor who opened St Christopher's Hospice in London in 1967, introduced the concept of 'total pain' (Saunders 1964) which encompassed physical, emotional, social, spiritual and psychological aspects of life. The idea of total pain became central to the multidisplinary team (MDT) approach of the modern hospice movement during the 1970s and 1980s. This idea of total pain has grown to include the consideration of the 'inner self' which is known only to the patient. This inner self is the person's own thoughts about what is happening in their lives and can have a positive or negative effect on their perception and experiences of pain.

Activity

Consider what you understand pain to be. Write down all the words associated with pain that you can think of. Now reflect on a time you might have been in pain. What made it better? What made it worse? How many of the words in your list have you experienced?

Consider your thoughts on distress. List the times you have seen a person in distress. What might have been causing this distress? What made it better? What made it worse?

NMC Domain 2: 2.3; 2.4

We return to the concept of physical, emotional, social and psychological aspects of caring for a patient in Chapter 15 on managing symptoms.

Affirms life and regards dying as a normal process

How can dying be 'normal' when a person is young, in a lot of pain or just retired and looking forward to the years ahead? This is one of the main challenges facing those who care for a patient in the palliative care phase. What we must consider is that from the time a patient is recognised as being in the palliative stages of their illness, it is important to support them to get a degree of normality. Thinking of ways to keep things normal is a really helpful way to support a patient and their family and can be a good way of building relationships and helping manage symptoms.

 Activity

Consider what a 'normal day' is for you. List all the activities you might do on a normal day. Now pick out three things in your normal day that are absolutely

vital for you. Now imagine you can't do these three things – how would you feel?

Now consider your practice placement and list the things that might impact on a patient's 'normal day': for example, visiting hours, times meals are served, number of visitors at the bed side, availability of a newspaper or access to the Internet.

NMC Domain 1: 1.1; 1.2
NMC Domain 3: 3.3; 3.4
NMC Domain 4: 4.3

Case history 5.1

A patient is admitted to your ward and, on the day of admission, he tells you that part of his normal daily routine is to walk his collie dog. He appears really worried and is very tearful. He tells you 'Since my wife died, she is everything to me and keeps me going'.

List the things you could do to support your patient.

(See page 50 for answers.)

Intends neither to hasten nor postpone death

As a member of the NMC register, it is essential to adhere to the law of the country you are working in (NMC 2008). In providing palliative care, it is important to balance managing distressing symptoms and ensuring our actions do not hasten the end of life. The terms 'euthanasia' and 'assisted dying' are often used in association with managing distressing symptoms and there is a lot of confusion about what actions we undertake and how these actions are not 'ending life' instead of managing symptoms and comfort.

We now consider the idea of 'double effect'. It is often thought that giving a patient morphine will affect breathing. Morphine is prescribed primarily as an analgesic, and in small quantities it can be used to help with breathlessness. A possible side effect of morphine is its sedative effect and sometimes this occurs as a consequence of managing pain or breathlessness. So there is a potential 'double effect' of giving the morphine. However, it is important to remember the morphine has been prescribed *primarily* to relive the pain and not decrease the breathing.

One of the challenges for healthcare professionals is to keep our personal views private while maintaining our professional practice. Understanding law and professional guidelines can help us do this.

Integrates the psychological and spiritual aspects of patient care

The word 'spiritual' comes from the Latin word 'spiritus' meaning breath, air, breathing. This idea of giving life underpins the definitions we have of spirituality and goes far beyond the following of a religion. Section 2 explores in detail different aspects of religious and cultural beliefs in order to help you understand how to meet patients' (and families') spiritual needs before, during and after death.

Understanding spirituality can help to care for a patient who might be experiencing distress. Psychological and spiritual care can be extended to a patient's family, both before and after death. A new concept in recognising and addressing spiritual needs is the work on 'Being' (Sheard 2007):

- Being.
- Enabling.
- Inspiring.
- Nurturing.
- Growing.

 Activity

In February 2010, the Director of Public Prosecution, Keir Starmer, announced 16 points of public interest for consideration to prosecute and 6 points to consider against prosecution. Familiarise yourself with these points by visiting the following Website:

http://www.cps.gov.uk/news/press_releases/109_10/ (accessed July 2011).

Now consider how you might respond to a patient who says the following:

'Can you help me to end all this?'

'If I was a dog, you would put me to sleep.'

'I am a burden to my family so I just want to die.'

Spending some time to consider how you might respond to these statements now can be a useful way to reduce feelings of stress when speaking with a patient or family about very sensitive issues. Write down some phrases that might be appropriate to respond to these comments.

(See page 50 for answers.)

NMC Domain 1: 1.1; 1.2

This work focuses on increasing our ability to 'be' rather than to 'do'. It originated from working with people with a dementia diagnosis, however it has some very important concepts which can be applied to any part of nursing care. The key ingredients of this approach are:

- *being* person centred
- *being* feeling based
- *being* self-aware
- *being* positive
- *being* supportive
- *being* congruent
- *being* together
- *being* passionate,

 Activity

In addition to the Being approach, consider the following definitions of spirituality:

'... the inner thing that is central to the person's being and what makes a person a unique individual ...' (Narayanasamy 2006:6)

'... is my being, my inner person. It is who I am, unique and alive. It is expressed through my body, my thinking, my feelings, my judgements and my creativity. My spirituality motivates me to choose meaningful relationships ...' (Stoll 1989:6)

What does 'spiritual' mean to you? Complete the following statement: 'As a spiritual person it is important to me that ...'

Now make a list of how you can 'be'. Consider how this might differ from 'doing'.

NMC Domain 1: 1.3; 1.5
NMC Domain 2: 2.4; 2.5
NMC Domain 3: 3.3; 3.4; 3.7

We are now beginning to see the links between physical wellbeing and psychological and spiritual distress. We refer to this as 'holistic care' and it is a fundamental part of the definition and practice of palliative care. Being able to understand the holistic needs of a person helps to plan care and reduce distress and is a fundamental aspect of providing dignified and compassionate care (McSherry & Ross 2010). We explore psychological distress in more detail in Chapter 15 on managing symptoms.

Offers a support system to help patients live as actively as possible until death

Here we think about a variety of supportive care measures to help a person be as active as possible. Ways of doing this include understanding how to manage symptoms and giving clear and concise information about what is happening and what is planned.

 Activity

Think about all the ways you can offer support. Make a list of the actions that you can do to support a patient to be active in their dying. Think of 'active' as something that can be physical, emotional, spiritual, artistic and practical.

NMC Domain 1: 1.1; 1.2; 1.4
NMC Domain 2: 2.1; 2.5
NMC Domain 3: 3.3; 3.4

Offers a support system to help the family cope during the patient's illness and in their own bereavement

When caring for a patient on a busy hospital ward or in their own home, it is important that their friends and relatives are given as much information and support as is appropriate. Information gathered in conversation from a patient or family at admission or from previous notes is a starting point. We now consider others ways to support the family.

When on your practice placement, find out the following:

Do family and friends know the nearest bus stop to use? Details of bus services? Where to get a taxi?

Will the visiting hours exclude a specific family member if they are working a shift pattern or a child at school?

Are flowers allowed in the clinical area? If not, do the family and friends know the alternatives they could bring in?

Who are the family members? Are they local or living abroad? One way of doing this is by completing a family tree or 'genogram' (Fig. 5.1). Have a go at writing your own family tree using the template given in Figure 5.1. It is important to keep each generation on its own line.

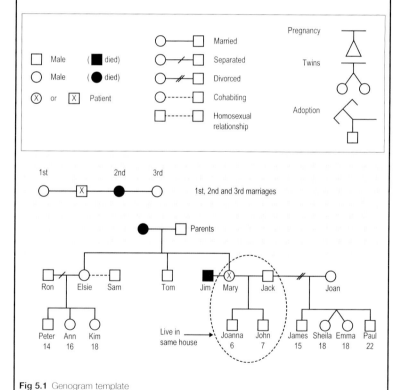

Fig 5.1 Genogram template

NMC Domain 3: 3.4; 3.8

Activity

If you want some more practice, complete a genogram for 'Mary'. The completed genogram for Mary can be found at the end of this chapter on page 50.

Mary is a 50-year-old patient.

Her mother is called Eva and is 80 years old.

Her father died 10 years ago from stomach cancer.

Her sister Eileen is 58 and has one daughter who is married with a 10-year-old son. She also has a son who is 30 years old.

Mary's other sister is called Joyce and she is 53 years old. She is divorced with no children.

Mary married Peter, however they divorced 15 years ago. Peter died 13 years ago and both his parents are still alive.

Mary and Peter had three children:

– James is 28 years old and he is married with twin boys aged 4 years. They live locally in Nottingham.
– John is 25 years old and he lives in Canada with his girlfriend.
– Lucy is 20 and currently studying at Leeds University.

After her divorce to Peter, Mary married John who is 54 years old and they have twin daughters – Ellie and Bethan – who are 10, and a son – Matthew – who is 6 years old.

John's mother died 3 years ago from cancer of the bowel. John's father died of a heart attack when he was 11 years old.

This is really important when things suddenly change and you need to offer extra support to family members. Knowing who people are and who is missing is a vital part of managing a distressing situation.

immediately after the death. This can leave professionals with a mixture of emotions. For some, not being on duty at the time of death can be upsetting. We continue to consider bereavement support in chapter 16.

Uses a team approach to address the needs of patients and their families, including bereavement counselling if indicated

Palliative care is not just about looking after a dying person but also the family at the time of death and into bereavement. Often in busy ward areas, the last time a nurse will have contact with a bereaved family will be when they leave the ward

Will enhance quality of life, and may also positively influence the course of illness

It is always important to remember that dying is still part of living and, as such, all focus must be given to ensuring patients' and families' needs are met at every opportunity. It is often the small things that make all the difference.

Reflection point

Consider how you might feel when you arrive on duty to find a patient you cared for has died. Write these feelings down.

Some things you can do to help work though your feelings in this type of situation:

Find out which team members were on duty when the patient died and ask them what happened.

Find out if family members were present.

Be prepared to talk through how you are feeling and listen to the experiences and feelings of others.

NMC Domain 1: 1.8
NMC Domain 2: 2.1; 2.6
NMC Domain 3: 3.9

 Activity

Make a list of the things that might improve the quality of a patient's stay in hospital.

Link these thoughts to the activities you have already undertaken. This list can be used when you first go to your placement area to help you focus on patients' needs in order to achieve a high quality of care. The list might help you to plan some of the outcomes you want to achieve while on the practice placement. These can be explored in your first interview with your mentor.

NMC Domain 1: 1.3;
NMC Domain 2: 2.2

The core terms used within palliative care

Having spent some time exploring in detail what the definition of palliative care means in practice, we now look at some common terms that are linked to palliative care, to avoid misunderstanding both by the healthcare team and for patients and their families. Some common terms you may hear used in your practice placement include the following.

Terminal care
This refers to a period when, despite the best efforts of patients, carers, friends, relatives and the multidisciplinary team, symptoms become more difficult to manage. The onset and duration of this period are as unique as every human being (Buckley 2008). There can sometimes be confusion about how the word 'terminal' is used and understood. A person can be referred to as having 'terminal cancer', making reference to the fact that the cancer cannot be cured, however they may have months or years to live a good quality of life. At other times, the 'terminal stage' is when a patient is in the last days or hours of life.

Last days of life
This is now a much more common term used and is potentially much clearer than the word 'terminal'. However, we must consider how this term may feel for the patient and family since it is much clearer than the word terminal, although more directive, and has the potential to be distressing. It is a term commonly used in current government and professional policy documents and training programmes.

Supportive care
Here we consider what is needed to help the patient and their family cope with cancer and treatment from pre-diagnosis, through

the process of diagnostics and treatment to cure, continuing illness or death and bereavement (NICE 2004). Supportive care can cover many aspects of care including financial payments and loan of equipment to enhancing comfort and dignity, counselling and respite care.

Respite care
Often a patient can be cared for by family members and neighbours very effectively in their own home, or in the home of a relative. However, sometimes there is a need for support that involves the patient going to a hospice or care home for a short period to allow the informal carers time to rest, go on holiday or catch up with paid employment or a hobby. Respite care is essential to keep the patient in their chosen place of care for as long as possible by giving support to carers. When a patient goes into a hospice or care home for respite, it gives the opportunity for their holistic needs to be reassessed and evaluated. Changes in treatment regimes can help with ongoing good symptom management.

End of life pathway
The End of Life Care Strategy (DH 2008) introduced the concept of a 'pathway' which would focus on the last year of life. This pathway is applicable to any patient diagnosis and helps health and social care professionals to plan ahead and ensure all the services possible are used to care of the patient and family. We return to this pathway when we look in detail at end of life best practice tools in Chapter 16.

Holistic care
Considering a patient and their life as a whole is the underpinning concept of 'holistic viewpoint' and is one of the foundations of palliative care. This includes spiritual, psychosocial and cultural factors as well as the wellbeing of family and friends. A patient can have their physical

symptoms well managed, but if they are concerned about family members, making a will or financial worries they may become distressed. So, in order to see the whole picture from the patient's perspective, we take the holistic approach. A patient experiencing a lot of distress associated with worries about family relationships is often referred to as 'existential suffering'.

Voluntary agency
This is an organisation funded mainly through voluntary money rather than through a government department. Some voluntary organisations are funded 50% by government money. It can be a registered charity and it may have staff in paid employment, as well as relying heavily on fundraising activities and volunteers. Some examples of voluntary organisations providing palliative care in England are Macmillan Cancer Relief, Sue Ryder Care and Marie Curie Cancer Care.

Activity

Access one of these voluntary agency Websites and explore the information that is available. Consider how much is relevant to the care of a person within the cancer and palliative care specialty. Follow through a theme you find of specific interest. Make notes on what you find out and be prepared to share this new knowledge with your mentor.

Macmillan Cancer Relief: http://www .macmillan.org.uk/Home.aspx (accessed November 2011).

Marie Curie Cancer Care: http://www .mariecurie.org.uk/ (accessed November 2011).

Sue Ryder Care: http://www .suerydercare.org/ (accessed November 2011).

> ### 🌣 Reflection point
>
> Reflect on what you think and feel about the palliative care definition. Is there any part of it you are particularly worried about or don't understand? Jot down your thoughts and use them as part of your first interview with your mentor to ensure your learning needs are met and you can achieve as much as possible from this practice placement.
>
> NMC Domain 1: 1.1
> NMC Domain 3: 3.4

Palliative care today

Consideration of the dying and the care we provide has gained a much higher profile in recent years. It became recognised as a medical specialty in 1987 leading to a new training programme for doctors to work towards becoming consultants in palliative medicine (Doyle et al 2005). Palliative care consultants have an essential role in the multiprofessional team and can be found in hospices and teams covering both acute hospital wards and community settings.

In 2008, there were nearly half a million deaths in England, though the main cause of deaths has changed over the last 100 years. This is due to a variety of reasons:

- Discovery of penicillin has reduced infections.
- Improvements in living conditions; housing, sanitation and water supply.
- Improvements in midwifery care leading to a fall in infant mortality.
- Improvements in factories and workplace safety reducing industrial accidents.
- More people living in large cities leading to changes in lifestyle: more sedentary workers having less exercise alongside changes in diet leads to more long-term

conditions, for example cancer, heart disease and stroke.
- Growth of hospitals and emergence of scientific medicine which can delay death, for example survival from a severe head injury.
- Emergence of special institutions to care for 'the dying' due mainly to the growth of the hospice movement.

In 2009, there were 220 hospice and palliative care units in the UK providing 3217 beds. Of these, 60 are run by the NHS and 160 are run by the voluntary sector including Sue Ryder Care and Marie Curie Cancer Care (Help the Hospices 2009).

Some of you will have a placement in one of these specialist units, while others will be applying the fundamental principles of palliative care nursing in a day-care department, acute oncology ward, haematology ward or an outpatient setting. Others may be providing palliative care in the acute setting of a medical or surgical ward.

In England, the Department of Health acknowledges the important role hospices and specialist palliative care have in the provision of care by suggesting they are the 'beacons of excellence in end of life care delivery' (DH 2008:10). The aim of this strategy has been to look at the main causes of death and consider examples of good practice across the country. It presents some core objectives to achieve high-quality care. These can be summarised as:

- being treated as an individual with dignity and respect
- being without pain and other symptoms
- being in familiar surroundings
- being in the company of close family and/or friends
- being given a choice and respected for choices made.

The End of Life Care Strategy (DH 2008) builds on the work of the NICE document *Improving Supportive and Palliative Care for Adults with Cancer* (NICE 2004) by linking these core objectives to achieving a 'good death'.

Reflection point

Spend some time considering what you understand by the term 'good death'. What would be important to you or for your family members? Can death be good? How do these reflections leave you feeling?

NMC Domain 1: 1.1; 1.2; 1.3; 1.8
NMC Domain 2: 2.5
NMC Domain 4: 4.4

When we consider what a good death is, we are thinking from our own personal viewpoint, beliefs, values and morals. This idea of morals links to the idea of ethical principles. We now look at what the term 'ethics' means.

The ethical debates in palliative care

Ethics is the science of morals, or human behaviour concerned with goodness and badness. Ethical principles are rules of conduct that can guide us in the way we behave, both personally and professionally.

In nursing, you will come across the term 'basic care' which refers to procedures vital to keeping an individual comfortable. This includes warmth, shelter, meeting hygiene needs and the offer of oral nutrition and hydration, relieving symptoms of distress by use of medication and comfort measures. Ethically and legally, basic care must always be provided, except where patients resist actively. In palliative care, the concept of basic care is central to decision making, as well as to the nursing care we plan and provide. Many practitioners worry that when a patient is declared to be dying, treatment cannot be given. Any treatment that relieves distress is appropriate.

The British Medical Association (2007:3) guidance to medical practitioners states:

the primary goal of medicine is to benefit the patient ... if treatment ... fails to give a ... benefit then that goal cannot be realised and the treatment should, ethically and legally, be withheld or withdrawn. Good quality care and palliation should however continue ...

One of the most challenging parts of treating a person is to know when to treat and when not to. This is hard for all members of a clinical team, even experienced doctors and nurses. Ethical principles can help us think objectively about making decisions in difficult situations. We will now look at 5 ethical principles, the first 4 were introduced by Beauchamp and Childress in 1977 (Beauchamp and Childress 2009). These principles have been expanded and developed over the years and remains a robust model today.

1. Respect for autonomy This simply means that a person has 'the right to be me'. Often, decision making can exclude patients in an attempt to protect them from distressing issues.

2. Beneficence This means to 'do good'. It is very easy to focus care on what we think is doing good when in fact it might be doing harm. Goodness is based on what patients want and need.

3. Non maleficence This means to 'do no harm' The aim in any nursing care is to do no harm yet sometimes harm can occur as an indirect consequence of doing good for the wrong reasons

4. Justice One way of thinking about justice is to think about how we offer a 'balanced fairness'.

5. Veracity This means to tell the truth. Sometimes a family may say to the professional team 'Don't tell dad he is dying as it will upset him too much'. What we must think instead is how we can support this patient *and his family* as he is coming to terms with his prognosis.

Activity

Will any of your actions do harm when they are intended to do good? List the range of nursing actions you may take part in on one shift. Now consider the potential for good and harm that might result from each one of these actions.

NMC Domain 1: 1.1; 1.2; 1.5
NMC Domain 2: 2.1; 2.4; 2.5
NMC Domain 3: 3.9

We return to nursing actions and explore them in more detail in Section 3.

Ethical reasoning

Ethical reasoning is an approach to working through doing good and doing no harm with the aim of achieving a balanced fairness. Ethical reasoning can offer an opportunity to discuss values and determine moral justification for a chosen action. Reasoning in this way gives the care team an opportunity to critically examine a situation by asking simple questions:

• What is happening?
• What went well?
• Why are we doing the things we are?
• What needs to change?
• Why?

Learning to question early on in your nursing career will help you to develop your skills in ethical reasoning and build the confidence to question care on an individual case.

 Activity

You are preparing to go on a ward round with the consultant and you don't understand a treatment a patient you have cared for this morning is receiving. Write down the questions you might ask based on the five ethical principles.

NMC Domain 1: 1.2; 1.6; 1.9

Final thoughts

This chapter introduced the definition of palliative care and guided your thinking to how you might deliver palliative care in your practice placement. One of the important elements in providing high-quality palliative care is to understand how you are feeling at any point in time.

Reflection point

As you prepare for your practice placement, take time to reflect on your current beliefs, knowledge and attitudes about palliative care. This may include what you have heard about the placement on previous placements, as well as experiences from other placements and personal life experiences. Consider how you might apply some of the principles in this chapter to the placement. Re-check your essential skills cluster and competencies and write down specific areas you need to achieve in this placement.

NMC Domain 1: 1.1; 1.2; 1.8
NMC Domain 2: 2.1
NMC Domain 3: 3.4
NMC Domain 4: 4.4

The wider concept of end of life care of which palliative care is a part is discussed in more detail in Chapter 16.

References

Beauchamp, T., Childress, J., 2009. Principles of biomedical ethics, 6th ed. Oxford University Press, Oxford.

British Medical Association, 2007. Withholding and withdrawing life-prolonging medical treatment: guidance for decision making, 3rd ed. Blackwell, Malden.

Buckley, J., 2008. Palliative care: an integrated approach. Wiley-Blackwell, Chichester.

Department of Health, 2008. End of life care strategy: promoting high quality care for all adults at the end of life. Department of Health, London.

Doyle, D., Hanks, G., Cherney, N., Calman, K., 2005. Oxford textbook of palliative medicine, 3rd ed. Oxford University Press, Oxford.

Help the Hospices, 2009. Hospice and palliative care directory. Help the Hospices, London.

McSherry, W., Ross, L., 2010. Spiritual assessment in healthcare practice. M & K Publishing, Keswick.

Narayanasamy, A., 2006. Spiritual care and transcultural care research. Quay, London.

National Institute for Health and Clinical Excellence, 2004. Guidance on cancer services: improving supportive and palliative care for adults with cancer: the manual. NICE, London.

Nursing and Midwifery Council, 2008. The code: standards of conduct, performance and ethics for nurses and midwives. NMC, London.

Saunders, C., 1964. Care of patients suffering from terminal illness at St Joseph's Hospice, Hackney, London. Nursing Mirror 14, vii–x.

Sheard, D., 2007. Being – an approach to life and dementia. Alzheimer's Society, London.

Stoll, R., 1989. The essence of spirituality 1989. In: Carson, V.B. (Ed.), Spiritual dimensions of nursing practice. W B Saunders, Philadelphia.

World Health Organisation, 2003. WHO definition of palliative care. Online. Available at: http://www.who.int/cancer/palliative/definition/en/ (accessed May 2011).

Further reading

Becker, B., 2010. Fundamental aspects of palliative care nursing: an evidence based handbook for student nurses. Quay, London.

General Medical, Council, 2010. Treatment and care towards the end of life: good practice to decision making. Online. Available at:http://www.gmc-uk.org/guidance/ethical_guidance/6858.asp (accessed May 2011).

Websites

National Council Palliative Care is an umbrella organisation in England, Wales and Northern Ireland involved in all aspects of palliative and end of life care. There is a range of publications, news updates and views from government, public and professional groups: http://www.ncpc.org.uk/ (accessed May 2011).

This Website, published by the UK Clinical Ethics Network, provides contact information for UK ethics committees, provides information on ethical issues and links to national policy and guidance: http://www.ethics-network.org.uk (accessed May 2011).

The National End of Life Care Programme Website has up-to-date information and publications on all aspects of end of life care and is a good starting point to search for local and national publications, polices and ways of working: http://www.endoflifecareforadults.nhs.uk/ (accessed May 2011).

healthtalkonline is a charity-run Website that shares patient experiences by facilitating them to tell their own story – many of these stories are presented in short film clips of 1–2 minutes long. You can choose from a variety of headings including receiving bad news, cancer and dying and bereavement: http://www.healthtalkonline.org/ (accessed on 7.5.2011).

St Christopher's Hospice in London publishes *End of Life Care* four times per year. This is a journal for nurses who want to deliver the best care for people dying at home, in care homes or in hospital: http://www.stchristophers.org.uk/ (accessed May 2011).

Dementia Care Matters: for more information on the David Sheard approach to meeting spiritual needs. This introduction starts with an interesting video clip: http://www.dementiacarematters.com/ (accessed May 2011).

Answers

Case history 5.1

Possible actions

- Find out who is caring for his dog while he is in hospital.
- Encourage pictures of his dog round the bedside, find out its name, encourage him to talk about it. Why does it have the name it does? How old is it?
- If he has a friend or family member, you might suggest one of them bring in a recent picture of the dog or, even better, a short video clip. Remember, some clinical areas will allow a dog to visit, especially if this is a hospice or specialist palliative care unit.
- The patient may also need to talk about who will look after the dog after he dies.

Activity

Some appropriate responses

- 'That feels like a difficult question to ask me.'
- 'Tell me why you have asked me that today.'
- 'I am listening, tell me more about how you are feeling.'

Activity

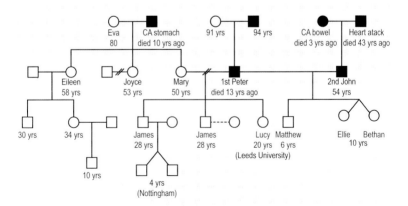

Fig 5.2 Completed genogram for Mary

6 Beginning the learning experience

CHAPTER AIMS

- Understanding how to prepare for the placement
- Knowing what to expect in the first week
- How to map one's own learning needs to NMC competencies
- Learning about the team
- Knowing the range of skills needed for the placement
- Understanding expectations of being a student in practice placement

Preparing for the placement

Each university will have its own curriculum expectations with regards to achievement of learning outcomes and assignment requirements. However, every student, through whatever practice assessment documents and processes have been developed, has to achieve the NMC Standards and Competencies in theory and practice in order to become a registered nurse. These combined requirements lead to an academic award (in future, a degree will be the minimum academic award to enter the nursing profession) and a professional award and subsequent nurse registration.

Earlier in this section we introduced you to some of the theoretical knowledge which will help you understand how and why individuals are diagnosed with cancer. This is important in order for you to start to plan for your cancer/palliative care placement. It is also vital that you reflect on your previous clinical experiences and consolidate knowledge you have gained in other clinical areas as well as in the classroom, enabling you to plan your learning objectives.

Before starting your placement, you should read your competency outcomes and essential skills cluster documentation and make a note of what your leaning outcomes will be on this placement. This will help you to start thinking how you might be able to meet these learning outcomes. It is important to do this ahead of time so you are prepared when you commence placement. This will ensure you maximise your learning opportunities and achievements. It will also demonstrate to your mentor that you have considered your own learning needs and are motivated, and this will be a good start at your preliminary interview.

As well as identifying the competencies you need to achieve, you also need to consider what *level of practice* is expected of you on this placement. This is generally dependent on where you are in your progression through the programme. For instance, as a first year student nurse, you will not be expected to work with minimal supervision, but as a final year student, this will be expected.

Although all student nurses are required to meet the NMC standards for pre-registration nursing education (NMC 2010) before progressing to registration, each university has a different method of assessing the *level* of competency. Benner's (1984) *From Novice to Expert* and Bondy's (1983) 'skills escalator' are examples of commonly used assessment strategies. Other universities may have an 'achieved' or 'not achieved' system. The NMC stipulated that this is not a sufficiently robust method and all pre-registration nursing providers will be expected to introduce a rigorous clinical assessment strategy, in which to measure the NMC Competencies.

Bondy (1983) (Fig. 6.1) uses four levels of achievement, and as students progress through their placements, they have minimum levels to achieve from 1–4. They can, however, meet a higher level in some outcomes or competencies if their mentor assesses they are working at that level. In each placement, they must meet the minimum level or the outcome/competency is not achieved. The levels are indicated in the ongoing achievement record on the corresponding 'assessment results' sheet for that semester. The level achieved for each outcome/competency should be recorded rather than merely a tick in the box.

Starting to develop your portfolio from the beginning of the placement is essential to ensure you are prepared for when you meet with your mentor to review and demonstrate your learning and clinical achievements, relating to the NMC Competencies and Essential Skills you need to achieve.

 Activity

Identify any outstanding learning outcomes from previous placements that you want/need to achieve, as well as the level of competency you need to achieve.

Refer back to the activities you completed earlier in this section. You should start collating all of this as evidence into your portfolio. This will help give you a guide as to which competencies you have achieved and which ones are outstanding, enabling you to concentrate on these.

NMC Domain 1: 1.1; 1.7; 1.8
NMC Domain 4: 4.4

Planning and preparation are competencies in their own rights and, as well as being essential to starting any new placement, learning these organisational and prioritising skills will be worthwhile throughout your training and in your professional role as a registered nurse. Levett-Jones and Bourgeois (2007) offer excellent advice and guidance for students prior to, during and after placements.

Roberts (2010) outlines key things you can do to prepare before starting a clinical placement. These include making sure you attend your planned clinical skills and simulated learning sessions and also, if an opportunity is planned into the timetable, undertaking some additional practice in the clinical skills classroom, either on your own or with a colleague (make sure your skills tutors are aware that you are doing so).

Practising skills prior to undertaking a placement can enhance your confidence when asked to undertake tasks that you have been shown how to do and may have practised a few times, but still possibly lack confidence in. Skills such as taking a blood pressure, for example, will be an essential

The Practice Levels below are the minimum levels of achievement for that part of the course. Students may be assessed at achieving beyond the minimal levels and should be encouraged to progress towards the higher levels

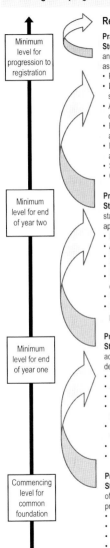

Registered Practitioner

Practice Level 4:
Student self-assessment: I have practiced with **minimal supervision** and within NMC and Trust Guidelines, meeting the standards of proficiency, seeking advice and support as appropriate to this practice level. **Indicators:**
- Prioritises care appropriately, demonstrating careful and deliberate planning.
- Demonstrates evidence-based practice approaches, drawing on a wide range of sources of evidence to support care delivery decisions.
- Actions underpinned with sound evidence-based rationales, communicated in a coherent and accurate manner.
- Demonstrates professional behaviour, showing awareness of responsibilities as an accountable practitioner in relation to self and others.
- Demonstrates ability to adapt behaviour/interventions to needs of client and environment.
- Safe, co-ordinated and efficient practice associated with an autonomous practitioner.
- Consistently communicates effectively with multidisciplinary team, users and carers.

Practice Level 3:
Student self-assessment: I have practised with **decreasing supervision** to achieve the standards of proficiency, requiring occasional support and prompts in the development of appropriate knowledge, skills and attributes. **Indicators:**
- Demonstrates increasing independence in initiating appropriate interventions.
- Applies knowledge to practice, providing a critical appraisal of the evidence.
- Makes informed judgements, considering more than one source of evidence.
- Demonstrates professional behaviour with underpinning ethical framework.
- Provides safe and efficient care under minimal supervision, demonstrating increasing confidence in own abilities.
- Gives informed rationale for care, demonstrating transferability of skills and knowledge.
- Communicates effectively with the nursing team and other health/social care professionals.

Practice Level 2:
Student self-assessment: I have practised **with assistance** in the delivery of care to achieve my practice outcomes (CFP) standards of proficiency (Branch programme) demonstrating knowledge, skills and attributes appropriate to this level. **Indicators:**
- Prioritises care and adapts to meet client needs with support.
- Applies knowledge to practice, identifying possible sources of evidence.
- Makes judgements, providing evidence based rationale.
- Demonstrates professional behaviour and understanding of professional responsibilities.
- Provides safe care under frequent supervision, demonstrating developing confidence in won abilities.
- Initiates appropriate interventions in relation to essential care without prompts.
- Communicates effectively with clients and the nursing team.

Practice Level 1:
Student self-assessment: I have practised, **with constant supervision**, in the delivery of essential care to develop the knowledge skills and attitude required to achieve my practice outcomes. **Indicators:**
- Undertakes care with direction and supervision from others.
- Identifies possible locations of information to support practice.
- Provides appropriate explanation in relation to care delivery activities.
- Demonstrates professional behaviour and understanding of personal responsibilities.
- Developing the ability to deliver safe and accurate practice.
- Initiates appropriate interventions with prompts.
- Developing communication skills.

Fig 6.1 Bondy skills escalator (adapted from Bondy (1983))

skill to learn if undertaking a cancer/palliative care placement, given the importance of blood pressure as an indicator of infection in an immunocompromised patient, such as septic shock.

Some universities also have excellent resources for students to use on their student learning Websites, accessible via personal passwords. You can also find useful resources linked to publication of books which also make a valued addition to pre-placement preparation.

A good example is the online clinical skills resource written by Docherty and McCallum (2009), available at: http://www.oup.com/uk/orc/bin/9780199534456/01student/checklists/ (accessed May 2011)

 Activity

> Log on to your own university learning resource centre (such as Blackboard) and find your online learning material with regards to clinical skills or preparation for practice placements. See the University of Nottingham for an example of practice learning pages: http://www.nottingham.ac.uk/nursing/practice/ (accessed November 2011).
>
> NMC Domain 1: 1.1
> NMC Domain 4: 4.4

A good way to dispel your fears is to make contact with your placement area. Many universities have placement details on the internal Web pages and this can be a good starting point for finding out about the area. Phone or e-mail the placement and arrange to speak with your mentor. You may use the placement checklist in Figure 6.2 to remind you of things to find out or do before starting your placement.

 Activity

> In preparation for meeting your mentor, check out the online information you can access about your cancer/palliative care placement, as well as the hospital or other environment where it is to be found. Check out the kind of treatment and care that takes place there and write out a draft plan of what you want to experience and learn during the time you are there. This could be a short placement within a larger placement learning pathway (or a 'hub and spoke' type placement) or a single placement where there may be opportunities to experience a 'snapshot' of a total patient experience.
>
> NMC Domain 4: 4.4; 4.5

Before your placement commences, enquire whether the placement has an induction/orientation package which will highlight the specific learning opportunities that might be available. Some universities will have these available on the Intranet before you start. In other schools, you may be given a pack on your first day or as the placement progresses.

An induction may include the following:

- Introduction to the placement and overview of the services offered.
- Chemotherapy and radiotherapy overview and safety features.
- Understanding spiritual distress in patients and the impact on the professional team.
- Opportunity to meet members of the wider multidisciplinary team, for example the chaplain and practice placement staff.
- Opportunity to explore areas of concern and personal feelings of anxiety.

Item	Yes	No
Checked dates of placement		
Found out where it is		
Found out best way to get there		
What time to arrive and the shift start and finish times		
What to take with me and where I can store my lunch and belongings		
What to wear (see uniform options) and where to change		
Name of mentor and Ward/Unit/Health Centre Manager/Sister		
Logged on the Course Learning Resource Centre (Intranet/password needed) and checked for any messages from programme/module leader/personal tutor		
Found out information available on any practice learning links on the school website		
Found out link teacher name for the placement		
Undertaken some initial reading about the kinds of patient problems you may come across and the possible care of patients		
Obtained a personal file for using at home to make notes on various health problems, signs and symptoms, medications, interventions, treatments and care, etc.		
If time, practice some skills relevant to placement in clinical skills lab with teacher agreement		
Refresh knowledge in any notes undertaken in lectures/seminars in University		
Obtain at least one book from library or other resource which is relevant to the clinical placement e.g. Corner & Bailey (2008) or Kearney & Richardson (2005).		
Ensure plenty of time to get to placement on the first day		

Fig 6.2 Placement checklist

Activity

Find out if this placement has an induction day. If not, use the above as a checklist to consider how you can prepare for the placement. You can refer back to this section to gather the core information.

What to expect in the first week

Once you have commenced your placement, there will be a number of key things you will need to know and achieve in your first day and your first week.

First day
- Ward layout.
- Fire exit.
- Fire extinguishers.
- Fire assembly points.
- Emergency practices.
- The location of the extravasation kit and cytotoxic spillage kit.
- Emergency call bell.
- Cardiac arrest trolley.

Within the first week
- Ward routines: visiting times; rest hour; protected meal times arrangements; meal times.
- What learning resources are available in the area: access to specialist resources; can resources be borrowed?
- Multidisciplinary team members in the clinical area: list their names and roles.
- Infection control policies: are flowers allowed in the area? What are the handwashing/rub facilities for visitors?
The first week can often be the most daunting and being prepared can reduce the feelings of anxiety, giving you more energy to establish relationships with team members and absorb important information.

Mapping your own learning needs to NMC competencies

You will probably be undertaking either a programme of study where the course is clearly divided into a 1-year common foundation programme (CFP) and a 2-year branch programme, or one where there is no CFP and branch evident but still requires a programme of study which enables you to achieve outcomes (NMC 2010) which are field specific (adult, child, mental health and learning disability nursing).

Regardless of which NMC outcomes you are having to achieve on this placement, the principles remain the same. You must adhere to both the *Guidance on Professional Conduct* (NMC 2009) and *The Code: Standards of Conduct, Performance and Ethics for Nurses and Midwives* (NMC 2008). It is very important that you read these and discuss them with your personal tutor before undertaking placement learning and also your mentor when you meet for the first time.

During your first week of placement you should sit down with your mentor and start to review your learning outcomes and identify learning opportunities in the clinical area.

Reflection point

Ask yourself the following questions:
What skills will be completely new to me?

What skills do I need to achieve?

Where do I need to add evidence to my portfolio?

What skills do I need specific practice in to increase confidence?

What skills am I worried about?

NMC Domain 1: 1.1; 1.5; 1.7; 1.8
NMC Domain 4: 4.4

Learning about the team

Establishing a relationship with your mentor or practice learning facilitator is important right from the first day. You should have been allocated a mentor and possibly a co-mentor and you should have your first day interview with one of them. Remember that the placement will have been informed when you are due to arrive and will have allocated you a mentor. Ward staff will be expecting you and will be keen to make you welcome.

As well as being supported by a named mentor, there will be a number of other qualified nurses (now known as registrants) and other healthcare workers and professionals who will help facilitate your learning and will contribute to assessing your knowledge and skills while on placement. It is important for you to consider the specific roles and responsibilities of these individuals. This is covered in Chapter 7.

Key roles linked to student learning in practice

The mentor

Every student who is allocated by their university to gain a clinical placement learning experience has to have a named mentor who will be their main facilitator of learning, supervisor and assessor of their practice (mandatory requirement of the NMC 2008). All mentors should be experienced nurses who will have completed a course of mentorship preparation or have an equivalent qualification in their own field which is recognised as being appropriate to supervise and assess student nurses in practice (this latter individual will only be able to undertake the mentor role in specific

placements and not at the major progression points within the new NMC (2010) guidance for curriculum delivery). Your mentor will be responsible for assessing your learning and competence in practice and your practice assessment document, as well as completing and signing your ongoing record of achievement (ORA) (Box 6.1), sometimes known as ongoing achievement record (OAR) (NMC 2007).

In addition to your mentor, more senior student nurses will take an active role in the teaching and support of other students as part of their role.

The sign off mentor

The role of the sign off mentor is to 'sign off' a student's competence against the NMC standards at the end of their NMC approved programme (Levett-Jones & Bourgeois 2007). This role is undertaken in the final placement only, but this decision will be influenced by the decisions of previous mentors who have recorded and approved the student's progress in their ORA in the previous placements. These mentors, as noted above, are critical to the assessment of the student's 'fitness to practise' as a safe and effective qualified nurse, and they are responsible and accountable for providing the evidence on which the 'sign off' mentor makes their final assessment. To be a sign off mentor, the qualified nurse must have undertaken a further course beyond that of mentorship.

As a student in the final placement, it is essential that you meet with the sign off mentor for the equivalent of 1 hour per week, in addition to the 40% of time working with your mentor normally. This is to ensure ongoing and constructive feedback is given as to your progress in that placement, and also builds on your previous ORA.

Box 6.1 Roles and expectations of you as the student and your mentor in relation to the assessment (ongoing record of achievement (ORA))*

The assessment process

Week 1

1. Student MUST negotiate with their mentor a time for their initial interview to discuss learning needs and goals and agree an action plan for achievement.
2. Student MUST share with their mentors their ORA from any previous placements and any action plans resulting from their last assessment of learning in practice.
3. Student will ensure that mentors are aware of any non-practice assessments they need to complete which may require their support for achieving, such as a client-focused assessment or evidence-based practice on a placement-specific topic.
4. Student may also have additional practice-based assessments to achieve in the placement, such as medicine management, handwashing skills or (ward/patient care) management.

Mid-point placement experience

5. Student and mentor will ensure that they meet to discuss progress at some point half way through their placement experience and also to determine if any actions from previous placement (ORA information) are being achieved. Evidence of progress will be gathered from a range of sources, including student skills record/practice assessment documents, other qualified nursing staff (registrants) and other health workers in direct contact on a regular basis with the student.
6. Student MUST receive constructive feedback from their mentor at this point and also on an ongoing basis. The mentor must ensure that the student is being taught new skills and gaining new knowledge through ongoing evaluation of learning and any deficit from their original agreed action plan can be re-negotiated if required. This mid-point meeting is an essential one for the student who may require additional support from their mentor to achieve successful completion of their practice assessment in this placement.

Final placement period

7. Student and mentor MUST meet during their final week of placement. (The importance of this final placement assessment will be critical for those students in their final placement as their practice will be required to be assessed by the 'sign off' mentor'). All evidence must be available about their progress on the placement and all documents available for discussion and signatures. Self-evaluation may be required as part of their practice assessment documents.
8. It is at this stage that the student has to offer clear evidence that they have achieved their goals, met the required NMC Competencies for the placement and a record made of their overall performance during their placement.

> **Box 6.1** Roles and expectations of you as the student and your mentor in relation to the assessment (ongoing record of achievement (ORA))*—cont'd
>
> 9. Ongoing record of practice assessment may either indicate level of achievement (such as the Bondy skills escalator, discussed earlier) as assessed by the mentor, or a simple assessment of:
>   - *Achieved*: all outcomes achieved competently, safely and professional behaviour appropriate.
>   - *Not achieved*: although some outcomes achieved, the student's overall performance has not met the required standard nor achieved required NMC Competencies for this placement.
> 10. Student and mentor discuss the outcomes and agree subsequent actions according to university policies.
>
>   *(Please note that this is a very brief version for illustration purposes only and that all universities will have different and very detailed practice assessment documentation.)*

Please refer to the full NMC guidance on issues of confidentiality and access to your ORA:

www.nmc-uk.org/Documents/Circulars/2007circulars/NMC%20circular%2033_2007.pdf (accessed May 2011).

The practice education facilitator

In some areas there are practice education facilitators; this is a relatively new role in practice education. These facilitators provide support for mentors and act as a link between mentors and colleagues in universities (Carlisle et al 2009).

Some practice education facilitators will work with mentors to develop supplementary learning opportunities for students in practice, such as student study days, workshops and shared learning opportunities with other healthcare professionals.

Practice education facilitators also work with mentors and link teachers/tutors from the university to develop and ensure that student placements are quality learning environments. They will also be involved in evaluation of your learning experience in the placement and also the educational audit, whereby a specific tool is used by the placement area to evaluate the quality of the overall learning environment to which you also will have contributed.

Link teacher

The link teacher role was introduced to strengthen links between education and service areas when nursing education was transferred into the higher education sector in the UK. Initially this role was key to the successful development of the learning environment in clinical practice, working with ward managers and mentors to develop placement learning opportunities and experiences for students as well as ensuring their quality. Of late, this role has become less visible but the link teacher still has a key role to play in ensuring that the areas which they link with support student learning (Arkell & Bayliss-Pratt 2007). You can check the identity of your placement link tutor through the placement learning information on your university Website and also when you arrive in your allocated placement.

The link teacher in many areas works closely with the practice education facilitators in ensuring good learning experiences for students, and some still retain 'hands on' clinical care and case loads. Some are also employed as lecturer–practitioners by NHS organisations, where they work half time in the university and half time in a clinical specialty (Buchan et al 2009)

It is important to make a note of your link teacher's name in your student diary because there may be a time when you need to contact the university directly, for example to speak with your personal tutor who may not be available and the placement link teacher may be able to help you instead.

The personal tutor

The role of the personal tutor is central to successful transition and journey through your specific field of practice (branch) pathway and programme of study.

It is expected that all students are allocated a personal tutor, normally from their own field of practice such as mental health, learning disability, adult or children and young people's nursing. Por and Barriball (2008:100) highlight that lecturers who undertook this role provided a range of activities from the 'provision of pastoral care and acting as a referral agent to other services such as student support networks, to monitoring student progress and giving academic support when required'. The main type of support that most students required was linked to these issues.

Your personal tutor will play a key role in helping you to achieve your personal and professional development goals or similar processes, which involves discussion of overall progress on your programme, including placement learning and achievements and academic achievements.

Activity

Discuss with your personal tutor what they consider their role to be and how you can ensure that both of you can work together with regards to achieving your outcomes during clinical placement.

Many universities will have specific criteria for the role and also guidance for what students expect from personal tutors and vice versa. Find out if your university/school of nursing has a document of this kind and discuss it with your personal tutor when meeting for the first time.

NMC Domain 1: 1.1; 1.5; 1.6
NMC Domain 4: 4.4; 4.5

Range of clinical skills available

There will be a variety of clinical skills including the essential skills clusters you can learn and become more confident in while on this placement. There will be opportunity to gain and develop general skills and experience in communication, decision making, leadership, nursing handover, discharge planning, referrals to other professionals and the ward round. These skills are transferable and you will take these into future clinical areas. They are revisited in Section 3.

Box 6.2 highlights some of the clinical skills you may undertake.

Activity

Pick two skills from Box 6.2 that you feel confident in doing. Consider what experience you have had that has helped this confidence.

Now pick two skills you do not feel confident with. Consider why this might be. For example, you may have witnessed last offices being performed by the nursing team, yet to feel confident you may want to perform this role. Or you might need to read up on the policy or have the opportunity to discuss specific parts of the procedure with your mentor or another member of staff.

If this is your first placement, consider what you have particularly enjoyed in your weeks of preparation in terms of clinical skills training. Now plan how you would pass this knowledge onto another person – this might be a colleague, relative or patient. Write down the key words and phrases you would use. Consider what you need to practise and develop competence in before you can explain it to others. This will help you to focus your mind on your key priority areas of learning.

NMC Domain 1: 1.5; 1.7; 1.8

Box 6.2 Clinical skills

- General assessment of the patient
- Prioritising planning and evaluating care
- Risk assessment: patient and environment
- Infection control
- Subcutaneous injection technique
- Asepsis
- Tissue viability
- Cannula care and extravasation management
- Care of central venous access lines
- Assessment and management of nausea and vomiting
- Assessment and management of pain

- Recognising dying
- Cytotoxic safety
- Radiation safety
- Observations
- Critical care
- Monitoring fluid balance
- Nutritional assessment (including body mass index)
- Enteral and parental feeding
- Administration of medicines
- Assessment and management of the oral cavity
- Moving and handling
- Last offices
- Complex discharge

Ways of developing your confidence

A good way of enjoying this placement will be to practise skills you already have; this will boost your confidence while helping you to consolidate your learning. For example, those who are towards the end of the training course will be able to teach first year students something new. This will provide evidence, for example, in your leadership and communications skills competencies. This will build up your confidence which is essential when you are qualified and working as a registered nurse.

Setting yourself goals like this with your mentor not only demonstrates your willingness to learn and your leadership abilities, but also helps you to expand your own knowledge and skills and consolidate previous learning.

Learning the terminology

Learning the terminology can be a challenge when starting in any new clinical area. A good way of ensuring new terms and

 Activity

If you are a senior student and undertaking a cancer/palliative care placement in your final year, before completing your programme of study it would be an ideal opportunity not only to learn to care for patients and their families in this environment, but also to facilitate the learning of less experienced students.

If you feel confident and competent to teach another student, agree a learning goal with your mentor to do this and, don't forget – make it 'SMART': specific, measurable, achievable, realistic and timely! (Fowler 1998:77.)

For example, you could teach a first year student nurse how to perform oral assessment or explain the World Health Organisation's pain ladder (Box 6.3).

NMC Domain 4: 4.1; 4.5; 4.6

Box 6.3 World Health Organisation's pain ladder

Specific – focuses on a very specific topic.

Measurable – it can be tested by question and answers to see how much the student understands about the assessment tool and process and by how the student performs the task.

Achievable – this is cancer/palliative care with patients who are experiencing different levels of pain. Explain to the first year student how the WHO ladder works. Remember not to over load them with information, instead relate the tool to a patient they have been caring for.

Realistic – you may have been given a lecture and participated in a seminar at university about teaching others, and if this is your second or third year you should have more than a basic knowledge of what is required.

Timely – it can be achieved in the student's placement experience regardless of length and you will be able to see impact of your teaching.

Activity

Identify skills and/or knowledge you have already achieved in previous placements. Consider how you might pass on this knowledge to someone else. Now imagine a patient or relative has asked you about a specific skill and think about how you would explain it to them. Write down some key sentences to prepare for giving this explanation.

If this is your first placement, consider what you have particularly enjoyed in your weeks of preparation or found particularly interesting. Now plan how you would pass this knowledge on to another person – this might be a colleague, relative or patient. Write down the key words and phrases you would use.

NMC Domain 1: 1.1
NMC Domain 2: 2.2
NMC Domain 4: 4.1; 4.4; 4.5; 4.6

abbreviations are not forgotten is to start to write them down in a list which is simple to refer back to throughout your placement. This will also help you to feel more orientated in your first few days

 Activity

Buy a small notebook for your uniform pocket. This is an ideal way to add to the list as the placement progresses. Remember: do not include patients' confidential or personal information in case it is lost.

Things you might add to this list are examples of diagnosis, treatment terms, common abbreviations, drug regimes and drug pseudonyms.

NMC Domain 1: 1.1; 1.5
NMC Domain 2: 2.7; 2.8

As you progress through the placement, your understanding of key terms and phrases will increase. This can sometimes be confusing and at other times be helpful in consolidating leaning. By writing down different ways terms and phrases are used, you will develop your wider understanding of complex issues across the cancer disease trajectory.

Expectations of being a student in practice placement

During your clinical placement you will be a *supernumerary* member of the team. It is important to understand what this does and does not mean. Being supernumerary means that even though your name might appear on the staff duty rota, you are not 'counted in the staff numbers' as being a member of the workforce on that shift.

Supernumerary does not mean that you do not become involved in *learning to work* alongside your mentor and other members of staff and telling staff in the placement that you cannot do something because you are there to only observe things. It also does not mean that you can come and go in that placement as you please! (You may think this is extreme and wouldn't happen – but it has been known.) You may, of course, come to an arrangement with your mentor in the placement regarding specific learning hours. Some placements, for example outpatient departments, only open 8–5 pm Monday to Friday; if that is the case then you also 'work' (or a better word is 'practise') within those hours as required by the university/school of nursing. Some students will also be in placement for only 3 days a week and then in university for the other 2 days, for example.

In addition to reading this section, it is important that you refer to your own university's guidelines and protocols as we can only provide generic guidelines.

Professional conduct and behaviour: Fitness to practice

In 2009, the NMC published its revised *Guidance for Professional Conduct for Nursing and Midwifery Students* (1st edition) with a further 2nd edition with minor amendments in September 2010. This new guidance is a very important document for all students regardless of any individual programme of study requirements or practice placement.

The full guidance can be found at: http://www.nmc-uk.org/Students/ Guidance-for-students/ (accessed November 2011).

 Activity

Sign up for the fortnightly NMC newsletter for up-to-date information on professional practice and student-related issues:
http://www.nmc-uk.org/Nurses-and-midwives/Have-you-signed-up-for-the-NMC-newsletter/ (accessed November 2011).

Another critically important guide for students is the NMC guidance on good health and good character (amended November 2010) which can be read in full at: http://www.nmc-uk.org/Students/Good-Health-and-Good-Character-for-students-nurses-and-midwives/ (accessed November 2011).

We hope that by now you are looking forward to this placement and feel you have really started to learn what it is about and what you might experience. Chapter 7 explores the cancer/palliative placement in more depth, helping to identify specific learning opportunities.

References

Arkell, S., Bayliss-Pratt, L., 2007. How nursing students can make the most of placements. Nursing Times 103 (20), 26–27.

Benner, P., 1984. From novice to expert: excellence and power in clinical nursing practice. Addison-Wesley, California.

Bondy, N.K., 1983. Criterion referenced definitions for rating scales in clinical education. Journal of Nursing Education 22 (9), 376–382.

Buchan, J., O'May, F., Little, L., 2009. Review of models of employment for nursing roles which bridge practice and education: a report for NHS Scotland. Project Report. NHS, Scotland.

Carlisle, C., Calman, L., Ibbotson, T., 2009. Practice based learning: the role of the Practice Education Facilitator in supporting mentors. Nurse Education Today 29 (7), 715–721.

Corner, J., Bailey, C. (Eds.), 2008. Cancer nursing: care in context, 2nd ed. Wiley-Blackwell, Oxford.

Docherty, C., McCallum, J., 2009. Foundation clinical nursing skills. Oxford University Press, Oxford. Online. Available at: http://www.oup.com/uk/orc/bin/9780199534456/01student/checklists/ (accessed November 2011).

Fowler, J., 1998. cited in Levett-Jones T, Bourgeois S (2009) The clinical placement: a nursing survival guide, 2nd ed. Baillière Tindall, Edinburgh.

Kearney, N., Richardson, A., 2005. Nursing patients with cancer: principles and practice. Churchill Livingstone, Edinburgh.

Levett-Jones, T., Bourgeois, A., 2007. The clinical placement: an essential guide for nursing students. Churchill Livingstone, Sydney.

Nursing and Midwifery Council, 2007. Ensuring continuity of practice assessment through the ongoing achievement record. Index Number: NMC Circular 33/2007. Online. Available at: http://www.nmc-uk.org/Documents/Circulars/2007circulars/NMC%20circular%2033_2007.pdf (accessed May 2011).

Nursing and Midwifery Council, 2008. The code: standards of conduct, performance and ethics for nurses and midwives. Online. Available at: http://www.nmc-uk.org/Nurses-and-midwives/The-code/The-code-in-full/ (accessed May 2011).

Nursing and Midwifery Council, 2009. Guidance on professional conduct for nursing and midwifery students. Online. Available at: http://www.nmc-uk.org/Documents/Guidance/Guidance-on-professional-conduct-for-nursing-and-midwifery-students-September-2010.PDF (accessed May 2011).

Nursing and Midwifery Council, 2010. Standards for pre-registration nursing education. Online. Available at: http://standards.nmc-uk.org/Pages/standards-download.aspx (accessed May 2011).

Por, J., Barriball, L., 2008. The personal tutor's role in pre-registration nursing education. British Journal of Nursing 17 (2), 99–103.

Roberts, D., 2010. Preparing you for clinical practice. In: Hart, S. (Ed.), (2010) Nursing: study and placement learning skills. Oxford University Press, Oxford, pp. 125–136.

Further reading

Aston, L., Wakefield, J., McGowan, R., 2010. The student nurse guide to decision making in practice. Open University Press, Maidenhead.

Davis, N., Clark, A., O'Brien, M., et al., 2011. Learning skills for nursing students. Learning Matters, Exeter.

Nursing and Midwifery Council, 2006. Standards to support learning and assessment in practice. Online. Available at: http://www.nmc-uk.org/Documents/Standards/nmcStandardsToSupportLearningAndAssessmentInPractice.pdf (accessed May 2011).

7 Placement learning pathways

CHAPTER AIMS

• To explore the cancer and palliative care placement
• To understand how each team/specialty works in the practice placement
• To understand the health and safety requirements in the departments that may be visited from the hub placement
• How to plan insight visits and opportunities as part of the practice placement

The cancer and palliative care placement

This chapter explains the varied roles that individuals, teams and departments have in providing services to patients and family members within the cancer and palliative care specialty. While you are on your practice placement, you will be working with some of these individuals and teams across a wide range of departments. Others may not be available at your local trust.

Although your own school of nursing/university and healthcare trust may organise your placements in different ways, many use the 'hub and spoke' model. Whether they do or not, this is a great way of identifying clinical learning opportunities. In addition to learning experiences in the *hub* placement, there are several *spoke* placements available as part of the learning experience. There are also potential opportunities to go on *insight visits* to work with multiprofessional team members, for example the community Macmillan nurse or escorting a patient for treatment in a different department.

These experiences are important to help you understand the role of each professional in the care environment and management of the patient and their family. Being familiar with the range of roles available and how they work in your clinical area can help in your assessment and care planning for a patient.

The 'hub and spoke' model in Figure 7.1 is supported by the NMC. It gives you the opportunity to be allocated to one clinical area for a period of time while also having the opportunity to be allocated to a spoke area and short insight visits.

In this model, any area could be either a hub or a spoke placement. Some teams

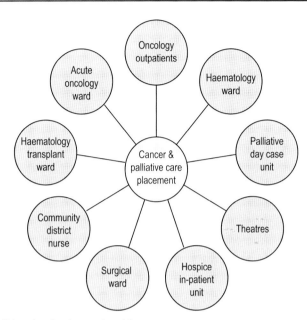

Fig 7.1 Hub and spoke placement model

and departments may be accessed by an insight visit. Your placement will most likely be composed of one hub with several planned spoke opportunities and insight visits. Discussing the opportunities available with your mentor is important at the start of the placement.

The length of the placement may depend on the year of study as well as local arrangements between the university and clinical areas. Box 7.1 outlines a theoretical example of what a first year nursing student's 18-week ('year-long') placement might look like. This sample placement demonstrates a wide range of learning opportunities that can stem from a core hub placement. It is important to remember that a cancer patient can be nursed in any clinical environment. Some placements will be much shorter than this, most ranging

between 8 and 12 weeks. This is dependent on the school of nursing and your stage of training.

These placement experiences reflect the patient journey and will give you some insight into how teams can complement each other with the work they do to provide holistic patient care.

Activity

You are allocated to a general medical ward as a hub placement for 8 weeks. Make a list of the spoke placements and insight visits you might be able to go to that will support the care of a person with cancer.

NMC Domain 1: 1.7
NMC Domain 4: 4.2; 4.4; 4.5

Box 7.1 A theoretical example of a first year nursing student's 18-week placement

Weeks 1–5: Hub – oncology ward

Focus on essential skills, professional behaviour and safeguarding. Observing cancer treatments: cytotoxic, biological and endocrine therapies.

Insight visits: radiotherapy, theatres.

Weeks 6–7: Spoke – oncology outpatients

Initial patient consultation, treatment decision making, follow-up clinics.

Insight visits: oncologist, site-specific nurse specialist, radiology investigations.

Weeks 8–10: Spoke – district nurse

Insight visits: Macmillan nurse, complementary therapist.

Weeks 11–13: Spoke – palliative day care

Insight visits: pharmacist, end of life coordinator, pain specialist team.

Weeks 14–18: Hub – oncology ward

Consolidate learning, reflect on the patient pathway.

Insight visits: dietician, discharge coordinator, occupational therapist, physiotherapist, social worker.

How each team/specialty works in the practice placement

The following individuals, teams and departments are potential spoke placements or insight visits within a hub placement. Some might be new to you while you may already have worked with others and understand their role.

Chaplain/chaplaincy

This could be a priest, pastor, rabbi, imam or another representative of a faith or belief serving a group of people who are unable to attend religious services or who need spiritual support and guidance. Chaplaincy is the term used to cover all these roles within a hospital environment. Chaplaincy teams can also offer support to professionals or teams working with complex or distressing situations.

Chemotherapy outpatients

This is a department which specialises in administering chemotherapy. It is staffed by trained chemotherapy nurses and is predominantly attend by outpatients. In some hospitals, inpatients will have chemotherapy in these departments.

Clinical trials team

Using evidence-based practice is important is all aspects of health care. Cancer treatments are complex and need to undergo rigid trails to test safety and efficacy. The clinical trials team are usually experienced nurses who will be working with patients and oncologists in the uptake of clinical trials and are responsible for the ethical and legal aspects of the trial.

Complementary therapist

This is a person who undertakes therapies such as hypnosis, homeopathy, acupuncture and massage (and many more)

that complement conventional medicine. Complementary therapists are often assigned to a palliative care day unit or hospice. Currently not all complementary therapies are available to all patients and there is a lack of national professional regulation. There are numerous qualifications needed to practise as a complementary therapist.

Cytotoxic pharmacy
This is a specialist unit where cytotoxic drugs and infusions are prepared in an air flow cabinet. Some larger centres will have a specialist cytotoxic pharmacist to advise oncologists on prescribing and treatment protocols.

Counsellor
This is an experienced counsellor usually registered with the British Association for Counselling and Psychotherapy (BACP). Patients and relatives are usually referred to the counsellor for psychosocial support. In specialist clinical areas, there is usually a counsellor as part of the team who will be on ward rounds and in the case conference.

Dietician
This is a registered practitioner who will advise staff and patients on the nutritional requirements for a patient. Their role is important in all stages of the cancer pathway, including advice to patients who have loss of appetite and taste following chemotherapy, for patients with restricted swallowing or with severe nausea.

Discharge coordinator
Efficient and safe discharge of patients needs to be carefully coordinated. The person in this role might be a registered nurse or an experienced nursing assistant or receptionist. Their role is to act as the centre point for the liaison of the discharge and they will link in with a wide range of teams, for example the district nurse, GP, outpatient department, ambulance services and pharmacy.

End of life pathway coordinator
This is usually a registered nurse who will be experienced in palliative and end of life care working within a hospital to coordinate the use of the end of life care pathway. It is often referred to as the Liverpool Care Pathway (LCP). The role will include training staff how to use the pathway and picking up specific problems with symptom management and support of relatives. Sometimes this role is delivered by a member of the hospital Macmillan team.

Haematological transplant coordinator/unit
This unit is a specialist ward for patients with a haematological diagnosis. Many of these patients will be nursed in separate cubicle and there will be strict infection control policies in place. In some hospitals, patients will be on a mixed oncology/ haematology ward.

Haematology day care
This is a specialised department for patients with a haematology diagnosis to come to hospital for treatment during the day.

Macmillan nurse or Macmillan team
Macmillan nurses are registered nurses with at least 5 years' experience who have undertaken specialist courses in managing pain and other symptoms and in psychological support. They work in both NHS hospitals and community teams. The role might initially have been funded (or still may be) by the charity Macmillan Cancer Relief. Many posts are now funded by the NHS although the title 'Macmillan' remains.

Occupational therapist
This is a person who has undertaken a course of study to register as an occupational therapist to help patients develop, improve, sustain or restore the highest possible level of independence through the use of activities or intervention.

Oncologist

This is a consultant who specialises in the medical management of a particular type of cancer by treatment with chemotherapy and/or radiotherapy and/or endocrine therapy and/or biological treatments.

Oncology outpatients

This is where patients go for a first appointment with the oncologist after they are referred by their GP, or return to see an oncologist/specialist nurse during their treatment plan. Many patients will return to oncology outpatients for years after treatment and cure in order to assess their wellbeing.

Oncology ward

This is a specialist ward where all patients with cancer will receive either treatment or supportive care. Some hospitals have several oncology wards while others might have some designated oncology beds on a larger ward.

Pain specialist team

This is a team of specialist practitioners, usually doctors, nurses and complementary therapists, who see patients with complex pain needs. The pain specialist team can visit the ward area or see patients in an outpatient setting. Treatment offered include epidural analgesia, lymph drainage or acupuncture.

Palliative care unit

This is a specialist unit for patients and their families needing palliative and end of life care. These units may be managed by an NHS organisation or a voluntary agency.

Palliative day care

This offers care and support to patients who live at home. It may involve symptom and medication reviews, providing hygiene needs, complementary therapy or social support. These day units are attached to specialist inpatient units or may be run by independent hospices.

Pharmacist

This is a person who has undertaken a course of study to register as a pharmacist. Pharmacists advise patients and healthcare providers on the selection, dosages, interactions and side effects of medications. Pharmacists monitor the health and progress of patients to ensure the safe and effective use of medication. Most medicines are produced by pharmaceutical companies. However, in the cancer setting, pharmacists may prepare cytotoxic medicines in a special sealed pharmacy unit in the hospital.

Physiotherapist

This is a person who has undertaken a course of study to register as a physiotherapist, who treats patients with musculoskeletal problems/physical problems in the main with exercise and other therapies.

Radiographer

This is a registered individual who takes images of internal parts of the body as well as undertaking some investigative tests – these include X-rays, computed tomography (CT) scans, positron emission tomography (PET) and magnetic resonance imaging (MRI).

Therapeutic radiographer/radiotherapy

This is a registered individual who uses MRI, CT and PET scans to plan and apply doses of ionising radiation (radiotherapy) or radioactive materials to patients in order to reduce or remove cancer.

Rapid response team

This is a team of experienced nurses who can be called to a patient's home to avoid a crisis admission to hospital. When a patient is discharged home, they may be told about the rapid response team within their area and how they can be contacted. It is primarily for patients at the end of life. These teams are usually based at hospices and specialist palliative care units and will work closely with the district nursing team and GPs.

Registered nurse

This is a person who has been approved by the NMC as being 'fit for practice' at the end of a course of study and who has met all the NMC Standards and Competencies for registration as a nurse. You will work with registered nurses on your cancer/palliative care placement in the inpatient and outpatient settings as well as chemotherapy, haematology, palliative and surgical day units.

Research nurse/research team

These are registered nurses who have undertaken a specialist role to recruit and coordinate clinical research trials. This clinical research will add to the body of knowledge in order to develop existing and future cancer treatments. The research nurse's role is to support patients while on a trial and to ensure quality of life is monitored and maintained.

Site-specific specialist nurse

A specialist nurse is someone who has a senior clinical role and has developed their knowledge and skills to an advanced level in a particular area of clinical care and offers additional expertise in the care of a patient. For example, a nurse may specialise in pain management or in a specific cancer, such as a lung nurse specialist.

Speech and language therapist

This is a registered practitioner who will advise patients who have difficulty speaking or swallowing, often referred to as the 'SALT' service/team.

Surgeon/plastic surgeon

This is a consultant who specialises in the surgical removal or reduction of a particular type of cancer, addressed as Mr or Ms. Some surgeons specialise in reconstructive surgery to refashion parts of the body after the removal of cancer, to improve the visual appearance or function. For example, they may reconstruct a breast after a mastectomy for breast cancer.

Social worker

This registered specialist offers social, emotional and financial support to individuals and/or families and liaises with other professionals to ensure effective discharge home from hospital.

Theatre

This is a clinical area where patients are prepared for surgery and given an anaesthetic, receive surgery and cared for after surgery is completed. Cancer patients may go to theatre for exploratory surgery to find a diagnosis or to have a primary tumour removed. Others may go for plastic surgery, to have a wound debrided (cleaned) or for insertion of an epidural or chest drain.

Ward sister/manager/charge nurse

This is a senior nurse who is responsible for the immediate management and leadership of a group of staff, together with overall management of the patients in their care. This will include clinical leadership in a specific field of practice.

This list is not complete and you may well have worked alongside or had some contact with a variety of other roles that support the care of a person with cancer.

◀ Activity

Pick out three roles from the above that may be new to you and find out about each one in more detail. Consider what you might learn from spending time with one of these individuals or in one of the departments and link it to your core competencies. This might be a visit you can plan at your first day discussion with your mentor.

NMC Domain 1: 1.4; 1.6; 1.7
NMC Domain 4: 4.6; 4.7

Reflect on your practice placement and consider if any role or specialty can be added. Maybe you have had a patient who has accessed a different service while you have been there. Jot down notes about this role and how the team on your practice placement liaised with this person/team. Consider how this enhanced the care and experience for your patient, family and your own learning experience. Also think back to lectures you have had. Write a short paragraph about this role that could, in theory, be added to the list above.

NMC Domain 1: 1.9
NMC Domain 4: 4.4; 4.7

Health and safety requirements in the departments that may be visited from the hub placement

For students who are not working on a specialist chemotherapy/radiotherapy ward, it is important to understand the precautions necessary if escorting a patient to one of these areas or if you spend a day in one of the departments. If you have attended an induction day for the placement, you may have covered these safety topics and this will be a refresher for you.

Cytotoxic medicines

Handling oral or intravenous cytotoxic drugs is extremely hazardous and this is not to be undertaken by a student nurse. Even if you are completing an oral drug administration round while being observed by a registered nurse, you should NOT handle these drugs. It is the responsibility of a qualified member of the team who has received training in cytotoxic handling.

Although you will not be administering cytotoxic medicines, you will be handling body fluids (urine, faeces, vomit) that may contain degrading by-products of the drug. In addition, if there is a spillage of cytotoxic drugs, you may be at risk if the correct procedures are not followed. The effects of exposure to cytotoxic drugs are irritation of the skin in the short term, the risk of developing a cancer, infertility and embryonic mutation (if exposure occurs while pregnant). However, these effects are *very rare* and usually occur in individuals who administer intravenous cytotoxic medicines all day, every day, for a number of years. By taking protective measures, the overall risk to your health is minimal.

Cytotoxic drugs are excreted in all body fluids but most of the drug is excreted by the kidneys in urine. The drug usually stays in the body for a number of days, but some drugs are slowly excreted, taking up to 48 days to clear.

While patients are undergoing inpatient intravenous cytotoxic treatment, they will generally be on a fluid balance chart to ensure their fluid balance is maintained. They will therefore be asked to collect their urine in either a disposable urinal or bed pan. The first principle is to dispose of the urinal/bed pan as soon as possible so that the urine left in a bathroom or lavatory can't be knocked over accidently (as well as for infection risk and hygiene reasons). Ask patients to use the nurse call buzzer when they have finished to ensure swift disposal.

Many cancer wards use absorbent granule sachets added to a bed pan or urinal before patients micturate. This ensures that the body fluid becomes semi-solid on contact and reduces the risk of spillage.

Note: before adding absorbent sachets, you must check whether a urinalysis (dip stick) is required. Some cytotoxics have side effects that damage the bladder lining, and all urine must be checked for the presence of blood to ensure immediate action to prevent severe damage. Also, before adding absorbent sachets, you should check if a specimen is required, such as a mid-stream urine (MSU) specimen. If one is required, take this in the normal way but label the bottle and the specimen request form with a 'hazardous waste' sticker before sending to the laboratory.

When you are ready to remove the bed pan/urinal, put on an apron and a pair of gloves and take the bed pan/urinal to the sluice. Once in the sluice, you will need to weigh the bed pan/urinal to attain an accurate volume to record on the fluid chart (making sure you subtract the weight of the bed pan/urinal and the absorbent granules). Then place the bed pan/urinal in the macerator (masher).

As well as body fluids, you may encounter a cytotoxic spillage. This is where a drug has leaked from either the bag or cannula or a urinal/bed pan has been knocked over. In this event, you will need to locate a 'cytotoxic spillage kit'. This should hold all the necessary equipment to clean up the spillage. As a student, you should not undertake the clean up, but may need to go and collect the spillage kit, so find out on the first day where it is stored. You may need to stay with the spillage, alerting passers by of the hazard.

 Activity

> Locate the cytotoxic spillage kit on your placement. Find out what is in the kit and read the local policy of how to deal with a spillage.
>
> NMC Domain 3: 3.6

Extravasation

One of the most common emergencies you may encounter in your placement is extravasation. This is where a drug (in this case, a cytotoxic drug) leaks from the cannula into the surrounding tissues causing damage. If left unattended, this condition can cause permanent damage and may require major plastic surgery to repair tissue damage.

There are many factors that may influence whether a patient experiences an extravasation:

Patient factors
- Number of previous cannulas or venepunctures.
- Very old or young patients.
- Confused, restless or sedated patients.

Drug-related factors
- Nature of the drug – pH, concentration, temperature.
- Amount of drug.
- Duration of exposure.

Healthcare professional-related factors
- Cannulation skill.
- Frequency of undertaking procedure.
- Selection of type/size of cannula.
- Selection of site of cannula.

To prevent an extravasation, it is essential that the cannula is secured in a manner so that the entrance can be observed. Many health trusts use guidelines such as the Visual Infusion Phlebitis (VIP) score as a way of monitoring and documenting the status of a cannula. Infusions should be monitored at least every hour, and bolus injections (where the drug is injected into the intravenous line) should be give very slowly through a fast-flowing drip. All intravenous lines should be carefully maintained and free flowing prior to any cytotoxic administration. The antecubital fossa should not be used, and any limb where sensory damage is present should be avoided. In addition, lymphoedematous limbs should be avoided, for example when a woman with breast cancer has had her axilla lymph nodes surgically removed and consequently the arm has become swollen due to the lack of lymphatic return.

Activity

How can you minimise the risk of extravasation? What are the principles of good cannula care? How might you recognise an extravasation? Does your trust use a VIP score?

NMC Domain 3: 3.2; 3.3; 3.4; 3.6

Have a look at The National Extravasation Information Service Website. Find out about the green card reporting system:
http://www.extravasation.org.uk/home.html (accessed November 2011).

NMC Domain 3: 3.1; 3.2; 3.3; 3.4; 3.6

If an extravasation is suspected, swift action is required. Cytotoxic drugs are categorised into groups depending on the damage they may cause if they extravasate: neutral, irritant and vesicant. The management of each type of drug that extravasates will be treated differently: either *spread and dilute* or *localise and neutralise*. Each department that administers cytotoxic drugs should have a policy for how each drug should be handled in the event of it leaking. Each department will also have an emergency extravasation kit which comprises all equipment needed.

It is important to know where essential equipment is kept, even if you are visiting a clinical area for just 1 day. Being able to locate items quickly is an important part of team working.

 Activity

Locate the emergency extravasation kit on your placement. Read the local policy, paying attention to the main methods of treatment: 'spread and dilute' or 'localise and neutralise'.

Look at a patient's cytotoxic prescription. Identify the extravasation category of each cytotoxic drug. How would you 'hypothetically' treat the patient if an extravasation occurred?

Radiation

You may be asked to escort a patient to have radiation treatment planned or to be given radiotherapy. It is important that you stand outside the treatment room when asked (or you might be asked to wear a lead apron) and that you adhere strictly to the safety requirements in the department. If you think you might be pregnant, it is important to tell your mentor or ward manager, in order for a risk assessment to be completed. This information will be kept confidential if you want it to be, but it is important that you protect yourself.

Obviously radiation has health implications, and ensuring you are not exposed to it is the key to protecting yourself. Every unit that administers radioactive treatment has guidelines called the 'local rules' that set out safe practice to protect all individuals. The key principles of the local rules of radiation safety are time, distance and using barriers. As a student nurse, you should *never* enter a room where a patient has a radioactive source within their body or is receiving external beam radiation (discussed in Chapter 13). Look for the radiation warning sign to identify potential patients. Where a radiation source can be removed temporarily (such as a 'selectron' machine), a qualified member of the team can switch the machine off. Once you have checked that the radiation has been safely removed, you may enter the room.

Activity

Locate the 'local rules' in your placement. These are set by the Health and Safety Executive and are implemented wherever radiation protection is required. Every area that administers treatment involving radiation must have a set of local rules.

NMC Domain 3: 3.4; 3.6

Planning insight visits and opportunities as part of the practice placement

As you prepare for this placement, having considered the wide range of teams and services available as part of the cancer and palliative care specialty, review your competency documentation and essential skills clusters and note down the areas that you need to focus on. Considering the spoke opportunities now might be a way of achieving a wide variety of competencies.

 Activity

Consider the various roles introduced in this chapter and the theoretical learning earlier in this section and start to plan what you might be able to achieve on this placement. Consider what you are looking forward to, what you need to achieve and what you may be anxious or worried about.

Now plan how you will communicate this in your first day interview with your mentor. This is a good way to plan the placement to ensure you achieve as much from it as possible.

NMC Domain 1: 1.5; 1.6; 1.7
NMC Domain 4: 4.4

This chapter introduced you to a range of individuals and team roles as well as departments within the cancer and palliative care specialty. Don't worry if you don't come across them all – you will certainly experience many of them and can then link them to the patient experience.

The next section focuses on the cancer/palliative care placement and identifies specific learning opportunities.

Further reading

Health and Safety Executive, 2003. Safe handling of cytotoxic drugs. Information sheet MISC615. HSE, London.

Nursing and Midwifery Council, 2010. Standards for pre-registration nursing education. Online. Available at: http://standards.nmc-uk.org/PreRegNursing/statutory/background/Pages/introduction.aspx (accessed May 2011).

Royal College of Nursing, 1998. Clinical practice guidelines: the administration of cytotoxic chemotherapy. Recommendations. RCN, London.

Wengstrom, Y., Margulies, A., 2008. European Oncology Nursing Society extravasation guidelines. European Journal of Oncology Nursing 12 (4), 357–361.

Websites

Cytotoxic handling forum and guidelines. http://www.marchguidelines.com/ (accessed May 2011).

The National Extravasation Information Service, http://www.extravasation.org.uk/ (accessed May 2011).

NHS Education for Scotland (NES), Website supporting practice education, with a specific forum discussing practitioners caring for cancer patients and the health and safety issues of cytotoxic drugs and radiation: http://www.nes.scot.nhs.uk/education-and-training/by-discipline/nursing-and-midwifery/practice-education.aspx (accessed November 2011).

Section 2. Placement learning opportunities

This section integrates theory into practice, highlighting specific issues involved in caring for patients at all stages of a cancer diagnosis and during a variety of cancer treatments and beyond. Specific learning opportunities will be highlighted and there will be activities, enabling you to make the most of your experience and to achieve your learning outcomes and professional competencies.

Chapter 8 explores the rationale for selecting cancer treatment and discusses some of the factors that influence treatment decision making.

Chapter 9 outlines the principles and advances in cancer surgery and broadly explores the care required when nursing a patient undergoing surgery as a cancer treatment, as well as the impact of surgery on an individual with cancer.

Chapter 10 outlines how cytotoxic therapy works, building on the cell and cancer cell biology covered in Section 1. It explores the practical issues in delivering this treatment, explains why patients experience side effects and outlines the care required by a patient undergoing cytotoxic therapy.

Chapter 11 considers the principles of haemopoietic stem cell transplant, which builds upon the knowledge gained in Chapter 3. Haemopoietic stem cell transplants are often very aggressive and frequently patients become critically ill post-transplant. The chapter identifies the care required by a patient undergoing this treatment.

Chapter 12 highlights some of the newer cell-targeted cancer treatments that are becoming increasingly successful and more widely used. It identifies some of the current biological treatments, as well as considering the priorities of care required by a patient undergoing biological therapy.

Chapter 13 discusses the role of radiotherapy, one of the oldest cancer treatments. Radiotherapy is often misunderstood by the public and it is essential that healthcare professionals have a sound knowledge of the treatment in order to explain to patients how it works and the procedures involved, as well as the side effects that they might experience. The chapter outlines the principles of treatment, as well as the care required by a patient undergoing radiotherapy.

Chapter 14 discusses the use of hormonal cancer treatments, otherwise known as endocrine therapy. The normal endocrine physiology is revised before an explanation of how hormones can be used to treat cancer. The chapter explores the care required for the patient undergoing endocrine therapy.

Chapter 15 introduces a range of symptoms a person with a cancer diagnosis *may* experience at points along the cancer trajectory as they move through a range of treatment options, as well as the potential to move into advancing disease. Recognising and managing symptoms is a fundamental nursing intervention and the chapter presents each symptom from perspectives of assessing, planning and evaluating care.

Chapter 16 explores the concept of 'end of life' and considers definitions, how to use best-practice tools and the application of core principles in a variety of cancer settings. A person with a cancer diagnosis may not enter into the end of life phase; however, it is important to be able to understand the impact of this phase on the patient, family and healthcare team as well as apply the principles of care. This chapter offers core information and tools that can be applied to the non-cancer patient and all the exercises are transferable into any clinical adult setting.

Chapter 17 considers the concept of life beyond cancer and how the transition from acute care into the follow-up phase may affect patients. It explores some of the long-term consequences of cancer and its treatment and discusses a few of the supportive strategies required by those living with and beyond cancer, enabling them to live a healthy and active life.

8 The rationale for selecting cancer treatment

Introduction

There are a number of treatments used to remove, reduce, halt the growth of a cancer or reduce the symptoms that may result from a cancer. The main treatments explored in the following chapters are identified in Figure 8.1.

Making a decision regarding which treatment to offer an individual diagnosed with cancer is complex and has changed over the past few hundred years, and especially in the past few decades, as knowledge and skills have developed. There are many holistic considerations to make to ensure that the decision-making process reflects the wishes of patients, as well as giving them the best possible outcome in terms of life expectancy and quality of life. The decision to use a treatment is influenced by the cancer itself, the patient, treatments available and environmental and ethical factors, all of which will be discussed in turn.

Disease-related factors

Over time we have gained a better understanding of how cancer cells develop, how cancer cells behave, why surgery alone does not remove all cancer cells and why cancer recurs. Each type of cancer has been studied in detail and we now have an understanding of the likely progression and outcome of most cancers. For instance, some cancers spread to distant sites very early; others very late; others never spread.

The size and anatomical location of the cancer may dictate the treatment plan. It may be too big to remove surgically or the position of the cancer may make surgery difficult. For instance, if the cancer is too large or is too close to a major or sensitive organ/tissue, the surgeon may not be able to remove it completely.

The type of tissue is important as some tissues are more sensitive to chemotherapy or radiotherapy than others. Therefore, the histology taken from biopsies is crucial.

Ethical-related factors

All patients have the right to make their own decisions regarding treatment and healthcare professionals must respect this autonomy. It is the multidisciplinary team's role to appraise all the relevant treatment

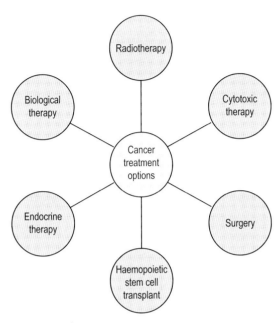

Fig 8.1 Cancer treatment options

options and the lead medical consultant's responsibility to present the options and consequences of each option in a balanced and unbiased manner. The patient has the right to information in terms that they can understand, at appropriate times, and the opportunity to ask questions in order to make an informed decision and consent to treatment.

Although most patients wish to receive information regarding treatment options and many want to be involved in the decision-making process in varying degrees, some want to make the decision themselves while other patients would rather the consultant decides for them (the patient may think the consultant has more knowledge/experience). Some patients feel that the responsibility and pressure is too

great; others feel overwhelmed by the trauma of a cancer diagnosis to make an objective choice; others want to be involved but view the decision as a joint decision between themselves and the healthcare team. No matter what their involvement in the ultimate decision, patients require tailor-made, accurate information so that they can make a balanced decision and give *informed consent*. Although the depth and amount may vary depending on the individual, healthcare professionals need to provide information regarding the type and extent of the cancer; what the possible treatment options are; what advantages might be encountered; and what the long-term effects of treatment might be. This information may need repeating several times and patients should be given an opportunity to ask questions. Encouraging patients and family members to write questions down helps them to remember what they want to ask about. Written information is particularly useful for referral at a later date.

All patients have the right to access cancer treatments fairly. However, in the UK, the availability of cancer treatments has not been equal for all patients. Prior to the Calman Hine report (DH 1995) and *The NHS Cancer Plan* (DH 2000), there was a great deal of regional variation regarding access to cancer treatments, quality of care and healthcare expertise. Each local health authority decided which cancer treatments would be available based on financial budget, immaterial of the effectiveness of drugs or the needs of patients. This resulted in spending variations, known as the 'postcode lottery', which may have contributed to higher death rates in some areas (although this was never proven). As a consequence of *The NHS Cancer Plan* (DH 2000), NICE was set up to review the clinical research trial evidence for each type of cancer and decide which treatments were effective and financially affordable. These two concepts are often in conflict and create ethical debate. Although there has been a reduction in regional inconsistencies and improved national access to research-based and cost-effective treatments, not all treatments are approved by NICE, and those that are approved are still sometimes unavailable and inaccessible by some patients.

Patient-related factors

The patients' level of education and previous experience in the health service may affect the treatment options as they may be able to comprehend more complex information, may understand the healthcare system and may seek alternative opinions. As well as knowledge, patients' financial circumstances may allow them access to treatment not available on the NHS.

Patients' values and beliefs about cancer and treatment may also influence their decisions. These may be based on previous experiences and beliefs. For example, a patient who is a Jehovah's Witness may refuse a haematological transplant, as this will involve the transfusion of blood products (Holland & Hogg 2001).

Although a patient's age will not necessarily directly influence the treatment they receive, the older the patient is, the more likely it is that they may have other medical conditions (co-morbidity) such arthritis, diabetes, etc., which may affect the body's ability to cope with cancer treatment. To measure a patient's general wellbeing objectively, assessment tools are used such as the Karnofsky scoring system and the World Health Organisation (WHO)/Eastern Cooperative Oncology Group (ECOG) score (Table 8.1, p.82). This is used to determine whether a patient is fit enough to tolerate treatment.

🔊 Activity

Select a patient that you are caring for. Look through their medical notes to identify whether they have had their performance status assessed. Discuss with your mentor how this information may have influenced the patient's treatment.

NMC Domain 3: 3.1; 3.2; 3.3; 3.10

In addition, an individual's situation or stage of life may influence their treatment choice. For example, if a patient considers that they have done everything in their life that they wanted to do or if their spouse is already deceased, they may not wish to undergo aggressive treatment. However, this is personal to every individual and healthcare professionals must be careful not to make assumptions. Just because a person may be considered older does not mean they have done everything they wish or do not want aggressive, fully active treatment. Patients' perception of their current and potential quality of life and projected life expectancy may also sway their decisions. Again, these are difficult to quantify and predict by the most experienced clinician, so must also be gauged carefully. It is therefore essential that a patient is supported to make an informed decision regarding their treatment.

Table 8.1 ECOG performance status (Oken et al 1982)

Grade	ECOG
0	Fully active, able to carry on all pre-disease performance without restriction
1	Restricted in physically strenuous activity but ambulatory and able to carry out work of a light or sedentary nature, e.g. light house work, office work
2	Ambulatory and capable of all self-care but unable to carry out any work activities Up and about more than 50% of waking hours
3	Capable of only limited self-care, confined to bed or chair more than 50% of waking hours
4	Completely disabled Cannot carry on any self-care Totally confined to bed or chair
5	Dead

 Activity

Visit the healthtalkonline Website to listen to stories of how patients' treatment decisions were made and how they felt about the process. The following link will take you to patients with colorectal cancer:

http://www.healthtalkonline.org/Cancer/Colorectal_Cancer/Topic/1070/ (accessed November 2011).

NMC Domain 1: 1.3; 1.4
NMC Domain 2: 2.4

Treatment-related factors

As well as financial resources restricting access to cancer treatment, treatment may be restricted by the experience and knowledge of the treatment team, the available clinical research trial results and the complications and potential mortality rates from treatment. A patient's previous cancer treatment may affect future treatment options. For instance, if an area of the body has already received radiotherapy then it may not be safe to give more. Similarly, some cytotoxic drugs have a maximum lifetime dose limit (Table 8.2).

In order to achieve the best possible outcome, patients often undergo several treatments (multimodality), highlighted in Figure 8.2. In most cases, the idea of this is to remove the primary cancer and treat any potential secondary metastatic spread.

The sequence of treatments can be done in several ways. Sometimes patients receive either radiotherapy or chemotherapy before undergoing surgery; this is known as *neoadjuvant* treatment. This approach reduces the size of the cancer, which may allow better surgical margins and/or better long-term functioning and/or better cosmetic appearance. Neoadjuvant

Table 8.2 Advantages and disadvantages of cancer treatment options

Treatment	Advantages	Disadvantages
Surgery	Gives good indication of the size and extent of cancer No carcinogenic effects May remove all cancer cells if localised	Patient may not be suitable for a general anaesthetic Possibly life-threatening (bleeding, infection, etc.) May result in change in cosmetic appearance and functioning Does not treat any metastatic spread Long period of recovery
Cytotoxics	Systemic – gets rid of metastatic spread Particularly good at destroying rapidly dividing (cancer) cells	Possible long-term side effects: in fertility, organ function Some cancers are not sensitive to chemotherapy Less effective with bulky, large cancers May cause cancer in later life Time-consuming for patients – repeated appointments May require repeated intravenous access or need for patient to self-medicate oral cytotoxics
Radiotherapy	Localised, therefore side effects only occur within the field of treatment Good for palliation of symptoms such as pain, breathlessness	Possible long-term side effects May not get rid of all cancer cells Some cancers are not radiosensitive May cause cancer in later life Planning is time-consuming Treatment is time-consuming If gonads irradiated, may reduce fertility
Biological therapy	Enhances the immune system Narrower range of side effects	Not suitable for treating all types of cancers Many are still experimental Possible severe allergic reactions May not get rid of all cancer cells

treatment is used particularly when cancers are positioned close to other major organs or where there is not a vast amount of tissue to take a clear margin, for example in head and neck cancers.

The most common sequencing of cancer treatment is *adjuvant* treatment. Surgery is performed initially, followed by chemotherapy and/or radiotherapy and/or biological therapy and/or endocrine therapy. This way, the main primary cancer is removed and then any possible metastatic spread can be treated.

Ideally, the goal of cancer treatment is to remove both the primary and secondary disease. However, if the primary cancer cannot be removed completely then treatment may still be given with the intention to reduce the symptoms a patient might experience and, where possible, to prolong life. This is known as palliative treatment.

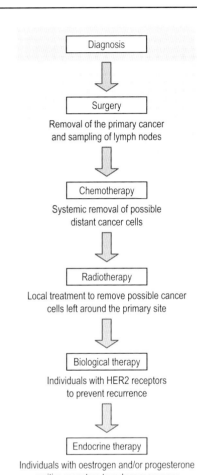

Diagnosis

Surgery

Removal of the primary cancer
and sampling of lymph nodes

Chemotherapy

Systemic removal of possible
distant cancer cells

Radiotherapy

Local treatment to remove possible cancer
cells left around the primary site

Biological therapy

Individuals with HER2 receptors
to prevent recurrence

Endocrine therapy

Individuals with oestrogen and/or progesterone
positive receptors to reduce recurrence

Fig 8.2 Example of multimodality treatment:
breast cancer pathway

Some treatments are experimental. These are known as clinical trials, and they test out new techniques, drugs and combinations to see how treatments can be improved or to find new ones. Patients may be offered a clinical trial at any point in their disease and they may or may not have any benefit from the treatment. There are different types of trials, known as 'phases'. A phase 1 trial investigates a new treatment to identify a safe dose, what the side effects might be and if the cancer shrinks. These trials involve a small number of patients and are often used once conventional/tried and tested treatments have failed. Phase 3 trials compare existing treatments against new ones to see if the new treatment or a different dose is better than the standard treatment in use. These trials are often *randomised controlled trials* (RCTs). In an RCT, patients are randomly split into two groups: one gets the conventional treatment, the other the new one. Sometimes patients do not know which group they have been placed in and they receive a placebo – this is known as a *blind* trial. At other times, neither the patient nor the clinician knows which group the patient is placed in – this is known as a *double blind* trial.

Although there is little guarantee in terms of treatment success for individual patients on the trial, and it takes many years before the results of a trial are known, some patients may benefit (physically and psychologically) from taking part in the trial. Clinical trials have transformed cancer treatments and symptom management as well as survival rates, and are essential to the future development of treating cancer.

Many patients you meet and care for during your cancer/palliative care placement will be receiving, or will have undergone, one or a number of these treatments. In addition, you may meet individuals with cancer in many healthcare settings who have a suspected or actual cancer diagnosis. For instance, while on an acute medical placement, you may meet patients who are being investigated for lung cancer, and on a surgical placement, you may meet patients being treated for colorectal cancer. Whatever the clinical environment, as a healthcare professional you should be able to explain how cancer treatments work and what patients should expect while on treatment, as well as being able to answer any questions patients or their families might have. This knowledge will also assist you to identify, assess and manage any side effects, ensuring you deliver high-quality, evidence-based care. The following chapters explore the principles of each of the following cancer treatments, identifying the possible side effects and care required: surgery, cytotoxic therapy, haemopoietic stem cell transplant, biological therapy, radiotherapy and endocrine therapy.

 Activity

Select a patient you are caring for who has been, or is about to be, enrolled in a clinical trial. Find out what phase the trial is in and what the trial is trying to find out. Is it an RCT? Think about the possible ethical implications of clinical trials. How do patients consent and what information might they need before agreeing to take part?

NMC Domain 1: 1.1; 1.2; 1.4; 1.9
NMC Domain 2: 2.2; 2.3
NMC Domain 3: 3.4

References

Department of Health, 1995. A policy framework for commissioning cancer services: a report by the Expert Advisory Group on Cancer to the Chief Medical Officers of England and Wales. Online. Available at: http://www.dh.gov.uk/en/ Publicationsandstatistics/Publications/ PublicationsPolicyAndGuidance/DH_ 4071083 (accessed November 2011).

Department of Health, 2000. The NHS cancer plan: a plan for investment, a plan for reform. Online. Available at: http://www.dh.gov.uk/en/ Publicationsandstatistics/Publications/ PublicationsPolicyAndGuidance/DH_ 4009609 (accessed November 2011).

Holland, K., Hogg, C., 2001. Cultural awareness in nursing and health care – an introductory text. Arnold, London.

Oken, M.M., Creech, R.H., Tormey, D.C., et al., 1982. Toxicity and response criteria of the Eastern Cooperative Oncology Group. American Journal of Clinical Oncology. 5, 649–655.

Further reading

Corner, J., Bailey, C. (Eds.), 2008. Cancer nursing: care in context. 2nd ed. Blackwell, Oxford.

Kearney, N., Richardson, A., 2006. Nursing patients with cancer: principles and practice. Churchill Livingstone, Edinburgh.

Munro, A., 2006. Decision making in cancer care. In: Kearney, N., Richardson, A. (Eds.), Nursing patients with cancer: principles and practice. Churchill Livingstone, Edinburgh.

Souhami, R., Tobias, J., 2005. Cancer and its management, 5th ed. Blackwell, Oxford.

Yarbro, C.H., Hansen Frogge, M., Godman, M., 2005. Cancer nursing: principles and practice, 6th ed. Jones and Bartlett, Boston.

Websites

National Institute for Health and Clinical Excellence, http://www.nice.org.uk/ (accessed May 2011).

National Cancer Research Institute (NCRI), http://www.ncri.org.uk/ (accessed May 2011).

9

Caring for the patient undergoing surgical cancer treatment

CHAPTER AIMS

- To introduce the student to the principles of surgery
- To understand the impact of surgery on the individual with cancer
- To explore the care required when nursing a patient undergoing surgery as a cancer treatment

Introduction

The majority of patients with cancer will undergo surgery of some description at some point and you may meet them in a variety of healthcare settings while on placement. Surgery may be used for diagnostic purposes; to get rid of the cancer completely; prophylactically (to remove an organ/tissue that may become cancerous in the future); for supportive care (enteral feeding, central venous catheters); to reconstruct a part of the body to improve functioning and/or appearance; and to palliate symptoms.

The success of the surgical removal of cancer and the impact of surgery has improved over the past century due to the following:

- Increased knowledge of the natural history of cancer biology and an understanding of how cancers develop and behave.
- The development of diagnostic techniques: this has increased the accuracy of staging and grading, ensuring that surgery is used appropriately and improves surgical outcomes. For instance, it may be inappropriate for a patient with advanced secondary disease to undergo surgery which will not eradicate the disease or offer benefit. More detailed diagnosis often reduces the need for radical surgery, reducing the physical and psychological impact as well as improving the overall outcome. A good example of this is the introduction of *sentinel node biopsy* (Farrant 2004). Previously, when a woman underwent a mastectomy for breast cancer, the surgeon would routinely remove some or all of the lymph nodes from her armpit. This often meant that women experienced long-term lymphoedema (swelling) and weakness in the affected arm. Now during surgery, the surgeon injects a blue dye (sometimes with a radioactive tracer) into the tissue close to the cancer. The dye drains into a number of the lymph nodes; these are then known as the sentinel nodes and are

removed to see if they contain cancer. If they are positive then the patient will most likely have a second operation to remove most of the lymph nodes under the arm.

- New microsurgical techniques such as laparoscopic and endoscopic procedures: these allow more conservative treatment, having less of an impact on physical functioning and appearance as well as a shorter postoperative stay.
- Since the Calman Hine report (DH 1995), surgical teams are dedicated to specific types of cancers. Surgeons must undertake a number of specific procedures a year to ensure competence, and all procedures are monitored locally, regional and nationally to ensure quality standards and equity.
- Recovery time in hospital has reduced as a result of the introduction of *enhanced recovery programmes*. These involve extra pre-, peri- and postoperative hydration and nutrition; regular analgesia; early removal of catheters/drains; and increased exercise soon after surgery (Slater 2010).
- The introduction of 'rapid discharge programmes' following surgery has improved physical and psychological recovery, such as the introduction of discharge after 23 hours from returning to the ward following breast surgery (DH 2007).

Prior to surgery, patients need to fully understand the procedure they are having. The healthcare team needs to outline the potential risks involved, the short- and long-term potential consequences of the procedure and possible complications. Gaining informed consent can sometimes be difficult if a patient lacks ability to comprehend often complex information – this may be due to a learning disability or a lack of education. The distress caused by diagnosis can often hamper an individual's ability to process information.

As healthcare professionals, we have a duty of care professionally, legally and ethically to ensure the welfare of patients. This may mean we need to act as an advocate, speaking on behalf of the patient during decision-making situations.

Activity

Read the article by Ford (2010) or Caulfield (2005) (see References):

Observe a patient being consented for an invasive procedure (this may be a central venous access device insertion or surgery). Write a summary of the main ethical, legal and professional aspects of accountability when gaining consent.

NMC Domain 1: 1.1; 1.2; 1.4; 1.5; 1.6; 1.7; 1.8; 1.9

The nursing role is essential in preoperative assessment and preparing the patient for theatre, both physically and mentally. Patients often feel positive about having the cancer 'cut out', but often have a lack of appreciation of the impact of surgery in the short and long term. Preoperative assessment should involve:

- medical history (co-morbidities and medication)
- functional assessment
- psychosocial assessment
- skin assessment
- nutritional assessment
- hydration/renal function
- pain assessment.

Depending on the type and extent of surgery (and the preoperative status of the patient), the patient will require a varying amount of postoperative nursing intervention to manage their airways, circulation, hydration, nutrition, elimination, tissue viability, personal hygiene, mobility and emotional status, as well as to ensure they are comfortable and pain is minimised. The multiprofessional team is key in ensuring an optimal rehabilitation.

 Activity

If you are allocated to a placement where there are many patients with cancer undergoing surgery, find out what preoperative assessment tool is used. Consider what the priorities of care are for a patient before surgery. How might a patient feel prior to surgery? Consider what the surgical risks might be for a patient undergoing surgery.

Read *Preoperative care*, Section 1 in Pudner (2010) (see References). Write a preoperative plan of care to meet the physical and emotional needs of a surgical patient you have cared for.

If you are in your final year of the course, then you might teach a less experienced student nurse how to prepare a patient for theatre or you might delegate an aspect of postoperative care. Remember, when delegating, you need to consider your accountability and what you need to ensure before delegating. Refer to the NMC guidelines:

http://www.nmc-uk.org/Nurses-and-midwives/Advice-by-topic/A/Advice/Delegation/ (accessed November 2011).

NMC Domain 1: 1.4
NMC Domain 2: 2.6
NMC Domain 3: 3.1; 3.2; 3.3; 3.4; 3.6; 3.9
NMC Domain 4: 4.6

 Activity

Identify a patient who has undergone surgery for cancer. Was the surgery the first treatment they received? Find out why surgery was selected. What is the impact of this particular surgery on this patient? Think about the physical changes: how might this make the patient feel? Will they have to make adjustments in their life? Is any further treatment planned?

NMC Domain 1: 1.1; 1.4
NMC Domain 2: 2.4
NMC Domain 3: 3.1; 3.2; 3.3; 3.4; 3.6; 3.7; 3.8; 3.10

 Activity

Revisit your lecture notes on wound healing. Summarise the main points and the most conducive environment for prompt healing.

Write a care plan of the immediate postoperative care required. Consider the importance of accurate and thorough documentation. Refer to the NMC (2009) *Record Keeping: Guidance for Nurses and Midwives*:

http://www.nmc-uk.org/Documents/Guidance/nmcGuidanceRecord KeepingGuidanceforNursesand Midwives.pdf (accessed November 2011).

NMC Domain 1: 1.7; 1.8
NMC Domain 3: 3.1; 3.2; 3.3; 3.4; 3.10
NMC Domain 4: 4.3

Often the team members will have introduced themselves to the patient preoperatively, explaining their role and what will happen after surgery. The speed of recovery will obviously vary enormously, but once the patient has made sufficient recovery and is deemed 'medically fit' and ready to return home, a comprehensive discharge plan of care should be in place to ensure rehabilitation and postoperative support. This is especially important in light of rapid discharge procedures.

With less time in hospital postoperatively, patients and carers are increasingly required to manage the consequences of surgery. To do this, they require clear, understandable, tailored information. This includes having the opportunity to discuss with their medical consultant the nature of their surgery and its progress prior to leaving hospital, as this will lessen their anxieties and provide much needed information prior to their post-discharge review meeting in the outpatients clinic (Mitchell 2010).

Prior to discharge, a referral to community services will usually be required to provide relevant care from the GP and/or district nurse. A follow-up appointment will be made for the patient to return for a postoperative progress assessment and to discuss the need for any further treatments.

Often, once surgery has been completed, an adjuvant therapy such as cytotoxic therapy or radiotherapy is planned. It is important that patients know what treatment (if any) they are planned for next, when the next treatment might occur and what they need to know beforehand as this helps reduce anxiety.

 Activity

Identify a patient who is due to be discharged home from hospital and plan the discharge by considering:

What rehabilitation do they require?

Are there any household alterations required before discharge?

Which other multiprofessionals need to be involved?

What information does the patient and their family need?

Is transport required?

What medication does the patient need once at home?

Are there any referrals to community services required?

Read the Royal College of Nursing discharge guidelines:

http://www.rcn.org.uk/__data/assets/pdf_file/0011/78509/001516.pdf (accessed November 2011).

NMC Domain 1: 1.3; 1.4; 1.5; 1.6
NMC Domain 2: 2.1; 2.2; 2.3; 2.5; 2.6
NMC Domain 3: 3.1; 3.3; 3.4; 3.5; 3.8; 3.10

References

Caulfield, H., 2005. Vital notes for nurses: accountability. Wiley-Blackwell, Edinburgh.

Department of Health, 1995. A policy framework for commissioning cancer services. Calman-Hine report). HMSO, London.

Department of Health, 2007. The cancer reform strategy. HMSO, London.

Farrant, A., 2004. A kinder way to stage breast cancer. Cancer Nursing Practice 3 (9), 12–15.

Ford, L., 2010. Consent and capacity: a guide for district nurses. British Journal of Community Nursing 15 (9), 456–460.

Mitchell, M., 2010. A patient-centred approach to day surgery nursing. Nursing Standard 24 (44), 40–46.

Pudner, R., 2010. Nursing the surgical patient, 3rd ed. Baillière Tindall, Edinburgh.

Slater, R., 2010. Impact of an enhanced recovery programme in colorectal surgery. British Journal of Nursing 19 (17), 1091–1099.

Further reading

Randle, J., Coffey, F., Bradbury, M. (Ed.), 2009. Oxford handbook of clinical skills in adult nursing. Open University Press, Oxford.

Rothrock, J.C., Alexander, S., 2011. Alexander's surgical procedures, 14th ed. Mosby, St Louis.

Wicker, P., O'Neil, J., 2010. Caring for the perioperative patient (essential clinical skills), 2nd ed. Wiley-Blackwell, Edinburgh.

Websites

NMC guidelines – Delegation: http://www.nmc-uk.org/Nurses-and-midwives/Advice-by-topic/A/Advice/Delegation/ (accessed May 2011).

Royal College of Nursing, 2004. Day surgery: Discharge planning http://www.rcn.org.uk/__data/assets/pdf_file/0011/78509/001376.pdf (accessed May 2011).

10

Caring for the patient undergoing cytotoxic therapy

Introduction

Many patients receive cytotoxic therapy as an adjuvant (after surgery) or neoadjuvantly (before surgery) so, although you might not be allocated to a specialist chemotherapy day unit, you will meet patients undergoing cytotoxic treatment in many healthcare settings such as wards, the community, hospices and outpatient units. It is essential you understand how these drugs work so you can provide information to help prevent toxicity and ensure prompt identification of any untoward treatment-related symptoms so intervention can be put in place.

Chemotherapy is the use of cytotoxic drugs in the treatment of cancer. It is a systemic treatment which means it travels to all areas in the body (other than the brain due to the blood–brain barrier) through the bloodstream.

Cytotoxic drugs work by disrupting cell division and act on highly proliferating cells

more than resting cells. The drug cannot tell which cells are cancerous and which are normal healthy cells, so the drug damages or kills both. However, normal cells have more ability to repair or replace themselves with new cells. This has great significance regarding side effects that patients experience, and knowing which normal cells in the body are affected can assist the healthcare professional prevent, minimise, assess and manage the side effects of cytotoxic therapy.

🔄 Reflection point

Recall the cell cycle in Chapter 2. Re-read this and determine which normal cells in the body are rapidly and continually dividing. Think about what specific impact this might have on the patient undergoing cytotoxic therapy.

NMC Domain 3: 3.2

There are hundreds of cytotoxic drugs, grouped together according to their biochemical nature (Table 10.1). We also classify the drugs in terms of how they act on the cell. Most cytotoxic drugs disrupt the cell cycle by damaging the DNA or affect mitosis and are classified into groups depending on which part of the cell cycle they affect:

- Cell cycle non-specific drugs kill cells whether in the cycle or resting, i.e. all phases: G0, G1, G2, S and M phases.

- Cell cycle non-phase-specific drugs only kill cells that are active in the cell cycle, i.e. G1, G2, S and M phases, but not G0.
- Cell cycle phase-specific drugs kill cells that are in a particular phase of the cell cycle, i.e. only cells in G1 phase.

Most cytotoxic drugs are given in combination – usually two or three drugs are used within a regimen. This enhances the effect of the drugs by killing more cells and minimising the range of side effects as well as lessening the risk of cancer cells becoming resistant. For instance, one cell cycle non-specific drug, one cell cycle non-phase-specific and one cell cycle phase-specific drug may be used. Each of the three drugs has different side effects which means the patient is able to tolerate a high dose and a greater tumour kill may be achieved if the drugs all have different modes of action. As an example, the most commonly used chemotherapy regimen for breast cancer after surgery is 5-fluorouracil (5-FU), epirubicin and cyclophosphamide (FEC) (see Fig. 10.1).

Table 10.1 Biochemical classification of cytotoxic drugs

Groups of cytotoxics	Examples of drugs
Antimiotic antibiotics	Doxorubicin
	Epirubicin
Anthracyclines	Mitomycin C
Non-anthracyclines	Methotrexate
	5-Fluorouracil (5-FU)
	Vinca alkaloids
	Capecitabine
Antimetabolites	Vincristine
Alkylating agents	Cyclophosphamide
Taxanes	Taxotere
	Taxol

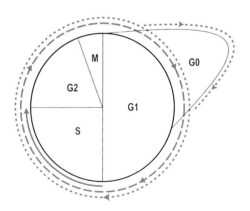

——— **5FU** - phase specific - only kills cells in **S** phase

— — **Epirubicin** - cell cycle specific - doesn't kill cells in **G0**

· · · **Cyclophosphide** - non cell specific - kills cells whatever stage

Fig 10.1 Action of FEC cytotoxic drugs on the cell cycle

Sometimes a single drug is used to manage or reduce a patient's symptoms.

Cytotoxic drugs and radiotherapy are sometimes given at the same time. This allows for both the primary disease and the secondary spread to be treated. Some cytotoxic drugs act as *radiosensitisers*, such as paclitaxel, 5-FU and capecitabine. This makes the radiotherapy more effective, however the combination of treatment increases the severity of side effects.

The timing of administration is important. Cytotoxic regimens are given in *cycles* – most are scheduled and repeated every 21 days over a number of months. This schedule allows normal cells a recovery period before the next cycle is started.

The FEC regimen mentioned earlier involves 6 cycles, each given 21 days apart. Sometimes, a patient's white blood cell count is reduced and does not return to the normal range at the end of the 21 days – then the next treatment may be delayed or *deferred*.

Cytotoxic drugs kill a percentage of cells rather than a fixed number, so the first few treatments kill more cells than the last treatment given. This is important if a patient requests to delay treatment. It is important that the early treatments are given to schedule, but there may be leeway with latter treatments (although this may depend on what the aim of treatment is).

Instead of being given in cycles, some cell cycle phase-specific drugs are given continuously. This is achieved by giving the drug orally or intravenously via a central venous access device (CVAD). The advantage of this is that the drug is constantly present in the blood and tissues. When each cell moves into the specific part of the cell cycle, the drug causes damage. Therefore, only a small number of cells are affected at any one time. For example, giving both 5-FU (intravenous) and capecitabine (oral) only damages cells that are in the S phase. A patient receives a continuous dose of 5-FU from a pump via a CVAD.

The pump contains 7 days worth of cytotoxic drug and the patient will attend chemotherapy clinic weekly to have the pump changed for up to 6 months. The 5-FU is constant in the blood and tissues and will damage/destroy any cell that enters the S phase. Because only a few cells are being killed, there are fewer side effects.

⟨•⟩ Reflection point

What might be the implications of being attached to a pump for 6 months? Think about the physical risks and the impact this might have on an individual's social/work life and body image.

NMC Domain 1: 1.4
NMC Domain 2: 2.6
NMC Domain 3: 3.1; 3.2; 3.3; 3.4; 3.6

Preparing the patient for cytotoxic treatment

Like for any treatment, patients must sign a consent form before they receive cytotoxic treatment. It is essential that they understand the reason why the treatment is needed; what is hoped to be achieved; what the potential effects of receiving the specific drugs are; and who they should inform if they experience any adverse side effects.

Before each treatment, the patient's individual dose is calculated using their body mass index (BMI). Height is measured on the first treatment, but the patient must be weighed at every treatment as they may lose weight, and some may gain weight.

A number of medical tests will also be carried out before treatment is administered. The types of tests undertaken are dependent on the types of drugs used and their toxicities. Blood tests, such as a full blood count, and biochemistry are checked to ensure the patient has normal parameters. Tumour markers (e.g. prostate-specific antigen (PSA) for prostate cancer; Ca125 for ovarian cancer; carcinoembryonic antigen (CEA) for breast, colorectal and lung cancer) are taken as these may be used as a guide to monitor the response to treatment. Depending on the type of toxicity, the following investigations might be performed:

- Creatinine clearance (renal).
- Audiogram (hearing).
- Electrocardiogram/echocardiogram (heart).
- X-ray and/or lung function (lungs).

Scans (magnetic resonance imaging (MRI), computed tomography (CT)) may also be done at the beginning, midpoint and at the end of treatment, to judge the response to treatment.

At each cycle of treatment, the patient is reviewed by a healthcare professional to ensure that they are tolerating treatment and the side effects are not too severe.

 Activity

> Find out how and where the cytotoxic drugs are prepared and how they are stored.
>
> NMC Domain 3: 3.4; 3.6

Routes of administration

Intravenous (IV) is the most common method of giving cytotoxic drugs as it is the most direct way of getting the drug into the bloodstream. However, there is the risk of infection and the procedure is uncomfortable. A variety of intravenous devices are used to access a vein: a peripheral cannula or CVAD such as a skin tunnelled (Hickman) line or Portacath or peripherally inserted central catheter (PICC) line. The choice of intravenous device is dependent on the quality of the patient's venous access; the length and frequency of treatment; the

potential risk of complications from a central venous catheter; the type of drug; and the expected need for additional interventions such as blood transfusions.

 Activity

> Watch the peripheral cannulation video at:
>
> http://cancernursing.org/forums/topic.asp?TopicID=74 (accessed November 2011).
>
> Find out which veins are used to site a peripheral cannula. What are the factors taken into consideration when choosing a site?
>
> NMC Domain 3: 3.2; 3.4; 3.6

Another common method of giving cytotoxic drugs is orally. The number of drugs given this way is increasing due to pharmaceutical developments. It is clearly an attractive method as the patient may receive treatment at home. However, it does result in less contact time from healthcare professionals which may lead to undiagnosed side effects and less psychological support (Irshad & Maisey 2010). There is the issue of concordance (compliance) – patients may not take the tablets as instructed, either forgetting a dose or taking too many. There is also the safety issue of storing medication in the home environment.

Cytotoxics can also be given intrathecally, injected into the spinal canal (via a lumbar puncture) so the drugs reach beyond the blood–brain barrier. This is used to treat patients with leukaemia. This is a potentially hazardous procedure as the risk of infection is high and there is a risk of spinal cord damage. Only three drugs are licensed to be given intrathecally and there have been several fatal cases when the incorrect drug has been given intrathecally instead of intravenously.

Cytotoxic drugs can be inserted directly into a bodily cavity, such as the bladder, pleural and peritoneal cavities. Cytotoxic bladder instillation uses a urinary catheter to insert mitomycin C into the bladder immediately after the surgical removal of bladder cancer. The bladder instillation is repeated intermittently for a number of weeks afterwards. Topical cytotoxic cream can reduce the size of some cancers affecting the skin.

Subcutaneous/intramuscular injections are very occasionally used. However, as most cytotoxic drugs are *vesicants* or *irritants*, causing severe tissue damage, and the absorption rate is unpredictable, these routes are not routinely used.

Side effects

Not all patients will experience untoward side effects following cytotoxic treatment. It will depend on the type, dose, scheduling/frequency of the drugs given as well as individual patient idiosyncrasies (some patients react in unexpected ways).

Many (but not all) side effects are either preventable or treatable so it is very important that we know which drugs cause which side effects so that appropriate measures can be put into place. Prevention of side effects is key and it is very important that patients know what they can do to stay well, such as: complying with taking medications (such as antiemetics); maintaining good oral and personal hygiene; well-balanced nutrition and hydration; and avoiding people with coughs and colds. Early detection is also vital to ensure a positive outcome. Patients must know what side effects to look out for and who they should inform if they suspect they have adverse side effects.

Patients often see side effects as an inevitable part of receiving cytotoxic drugs and think that they must endure and tolerate them. As a result, some patients are reluctant to report side effects as they fear that treatment may be withdrawn, thus reducing the success. It is often difficult for patients to interpret the significance/severity of side effects and know when to seek advice. For instance, they might think that pins and needles might be due to a trapped nerve rather than a neurological toxicity of a cytotoxic (Table 10.2).

Table 10.2 Common toxicities of cytotoxic drugs	
Seconds/ minutes	Allergic reactions, flushing, nausea, taste alteration
Days/ weeks	Mucositis, nausea and vomiting (acute, delayed, anticipatory), alopecia, diarrhoea, neutropenia, thrombocytopenia
Months/ years	Anaemia, neurological, organ toxicity (heart, lung, liver, kidney), secondary tumours

 Activity

Identify a patient undergoing cytotoxic therapy. Ask what side effects they have experienced. Then look up the relevant cytotoxic drugs – what are the common side effects caused by these drugs specifically? Does the patient's experience reflect the expected side effects?

Keep a note of the name of the drug(s), mode of action and side effects in your notebook for future reference.

NMC Domain 1: 1.4
NMC Domain 2: 2.3
NMC Domain 3: 3.1; 3.3; 3.6; 3.7

Cytotoxic-induced nausea and vomiting

Cytotoxic drugs damage the rapidly dividing cells that line the gastrointestinal tract resulting in nausea and vomiting. In addition, the chemoreceptor trigger zone (CTZ) in the brain is stimulated, registering that there are toxic substances in the body. Cytotoxic-induced nausea and vomiting (CINV) is reported as one of the most distressing side effects of treatment (Bergkvist & Wengstrom 2006), with approximately 50% of patients experiencing nausea and/or vomiting, resulting in significant distress (Molassiotis et al 2008).

CINV can easily be prevented using appropriate antiemetics (anti-sickness) drugs which are usually given at the same time as the cytotoxic treatment and for a number of days afterwards. Each cytotoxic drug has been graded in terms of its emetogenic property, some causing severe CINV, others very little. Each regimen has a standard antiemetic protocol, usually a combination of antiemetics, although this may differ slightly in each hospital. If a patient experiences CINV despite receiving the antiemetic protocol, then additional or alternative antiemetics are used. Some individuals are more susceptible to CINV, such as women, those who experience travel sickness, those who have a low consumption of alcohol and those who experience antenatal nausea and vomiting.

Anticipatory nausea and vomiting is a distressing condition resulting from a psychological reaction to cytotoxic treatment. It usually develops over time and the patient associates a traumatic feeling with the hospital environment, a specific nurse or a cannula. This becomes overwhelming and is expressed as nausea and vomiting. Because this is caused by an emotional rather than a physiological reaction, it is not responsive to antiemetics. Instead, non-pharmacological therapy, such as hypnotherapy and visualisation techniques, may be helpful. Nausea and vomiting is explored further in Chapter 15.

 Activity

> Find out about the most common antiemetic drugs used to prevent and manage cytotoxic-induced nausea and vomiting. Which part(s) of the body do these drugs act upon?
>
> NMC Domain 1: 1.7; 1.9
> NMC Domain 3: 3.1; 3.2

Alopecia

Eighty-five per cent of hair follicles are actively in the cell cycle (this is why hair continually grows). Therefore, hair loss is a common side effect of cytotoxic treatment, especially when the drugs are cell cycle non-specific (killing more cells off in one go). It normally takes a month or two before the hair begins to come out in a noticeable amount, but after a couple of weeks the patient will find more hair in the plug hole after washing their hair and in the hairbrush. The more a patient styles or handles their hair, the quicker it will come out. Washing with a 'frequent wash' shampoo will help prolong the process, however eventually there will be complete loss. This is often extremely distressing for patients, affecting their body image and sexuality (Power & Condon 2008).

Scalp cooling is a way of trying to minimise hair loss by reducing the temperature of the scalp and restricting the blood flow to the hair follicles, thus reducing the amount of cytotoxic drug reaching the follicle and damaging the cell. There are several ways of cooling the scalp – the most common is using a cold cap that is filled with gel and then chilled. The cap fits closely to the scalp and is worn for half the time it takes for the body to get rid of the drug. In addition, the cap requires changing as it warms up. This means that scalp cooling can only be used for a small number of patients who are receiving cytotoxic therapy administered over a short period of time, with a short half-life. For example, with the FEC regimen (mentioned above), a normal treatment time is approximately 45 minutes in total. When using scalp cooling, the cannula is placed first and a cold cap is worn for 15 minutes. This is then replaced by another cap and treatment is commenced. After 45 minutes, the cap is replaced and worn for a further 45 minutes, a total of 1 hour and 45 minutes, more than doubling treatment time. Scalp cooling does not prevent hair loss – it is just a way of retaining some hair and often it is not successful. After treatment, hair will return but this may take a number of months. Also, the hair may return a different colour or texture (Van den Hurk et al 2010).

 Activity

Find out which method of scalp cooling is used in your practice area. Observe it in action and consider the effects and benefits experienced by the patient. If this treatment is not available on your placement, find out where it is available and plan an 'insight visit' or spoke placement visit to that area.

NMC Domain 3: 3.4; 3.6

Neutropenia

Neutropenia, sometimes known as *immunosupression*, is the most life-threatening side effect of receiving cytotoxic treatment. As well as causing direct mortality, neutropenia may delay treatment, reducing the overall efficacy of cytotoxics (Methven 2010). Neutropenia-related infections result in additional hospital admissions and impact on patients' quality of life.

Neutropenia occurs when the number of neutrophils in the blood drops below 1×10^9/L. A normal range of neutrophils is 2.5–7.5 $\times 10^9$/L. We concentrate on neutrophils rather than white blood cells overall, as they are the type of white blood cells we have the most of (70% of white blood cells are neutrophils). They are also our first line of defence – being phagocytes, they ingest microorganisms or pathogens (bacteria, fungi or viruses).

Stem cells take 3 days to produce a neutrophil, before releasing it into the peripheral blood where it lives for 7 hours. Because of this long process of making a neutrophil and its short life span, the bone marrow is continually making neutrophils. Cytotoxic drugs kill/damage the neutrophils in the peripheral blood and the stem cells in the bone marrow. It takes an average of 7–10 days for a patient to become neutropenic and to reach the *nadir* (the lowest point). This is the time when the patient is most at risk from infection.

Individuals with a cancer diagnosis are at high risk of infection not only due to the effects of cytotoxic drugs, but also to the number of invasive procedures they undergo. Many medications they receive, such as steroids, increase the risk. As discussed in Section 1, cancer generally occurs in older individuals. As we get older, our immune system is less effective and there is increased likelihood of other co-morbidity, such as diabetes. This will increase the risk of infection.

 Activity

Re-read your lecture notes or an anatomy and physiology textbook (such as to refresh your knowledge of the body's immune response to infection. Read Coughlan and Healey (2008) (see References for details) for more information about caring for patients with neutropenia.

Make a list of factors that may influence the risk of infection in cancer patients.

NMC Domain 3: 3.1; 3.2; 3.3; 3.4; 3.7; 3.8; 3.10

When a patient is neutropenic, many *endogenous* pathogens living in the patient's body (normally not doing any harm) are able to use the opportunity of the reduced immune system to cause damage (Vento & Cainelli 2003). A good example of this is the *herpes simplex virus*, otherwise known as a cold sore. We may never know how or when we became infected by the virus, but as soon as we are feeling run down or are getting over an illness, the virus can activate and develop in a lesion, usually on the lip. Another example is the *varicella zoster virus*, otherwise known as chickenpox. A patient may have had chickenpox as a small child – although they recover from the spots and fever, the virus remains in the body in a dormant state in the nerve tissues. It reactivates when the immune system is low or working especially hard; this is known as *shingles*. Shingles can be extremely painful and cause respiratory damage. In an immunosuppressed patient, it may be fatal.

Infections from external or *exogenous* sources can also cause harm. Effective hand washing is essential for the patient, family and healthcare professionals. Patients should also avoid contact with anyone with infections, like a cough or cold.

All patients undergoing cytotoxic therapy should take their temperature daily (at a similar time of day) and should be kept at home to avoid hospital-acquired infections. However, if they become pyrexial (temperature aboe 37.5°C on more than two occasions or 38°C on one occasion), they should telephone the chemotherapy unit urgently. Not all patients with an infection have a temperature, so if they feel unwell they should also phone the chemotherapy unit for advice.

Patients undergoing cytotoxic treatment should avoid taking paracetamol (Coughlan & Healey 2008). This is because having a temperature or pyrexia helps the body to mount an immune response to fight the pathogen in the body. A temperature acts as a signal to the immune system/white blood cells to go to the site of infection and kill the invader. Paracetamol artificially reduces body temperature by 'resetting' the hypothalamus (like a thermostat). This indicates to the immune system there isn't a problem. When the temperature is within the normal range, the patient or healthcare professional may think that there is no longer a problem and not respond. If the cause of the infection is not treated then the patient may become septic and go into shock and may suffer a cardiac arrest. Therefore, it is vital that the early signs and symptoms of infection are detected and prompt action is taken.

Activity

Make a list of the signs and symptoms of infection. How will you assess a patient with suspected neutropenic sepsis?

Watch the neutropenic sepsis video on the Cancer Nursing Website: http://cancernursing.org/forums/topic.asp?TopicID=100 (accessed November 2011).

Find out what the neutropenic policy and protocol are in your area. Discuss any issues that you are not sure about with your mentor.

NMC Domain 3: 3.1; 3.2; 3.3; 3.4; 3.7; 3.8; 3.10

Mucositis

Because the mucosa (lining of the oral cavity) is continually renewing itself, it is very sensitive to cytotoxic drugs. Approximately 40% of patients undergoing cytotoxic therapy will develop *mucositis*, sometimes known as *stomatitis* (Raber-Durlacher et al 2010). This can affect a patient's nutritional status, communication and body image, and may cause pain.

Treatment may be halted or postponed, particularly if the mucositis is severe. The effect can be minimised by regular teeth cleaning after each meal. No special mouth washes are required (Van Achterberg 2007). Ice chips help reduce the chance of mucositis, by reducing the blood supply and slowing the cell cycle of the cells lining the mouth (Nikoletti et al 2005, Worthington et al 2006).

Other side effects

Taste alteration (often metallic) is common while cytotoxic drugs are being infused, and may affect a patient's appetite. This can be improved by sucking boiled sweets.

There are no particular diet restrictions for patients undergoing chemotherapy, however shellfish, raw eggs and unpasteurised dairy should be avoided to minimise the risk of infection (Brown 2010).

In the long term, cytotoxic drugs may cause a second cancer to develop, as a result of the damage done to the DNA, patients should be informed of this when consenting for treatment.

Summary

Although patients may receive verbal and written information regarding what to expect in the way of side effects, they may not be able to interpret signs and symptoms or may be worried about reporting problems in case treatment is reduced or withdrawn. It is important that patients report adverse effects in order to manage these problems. If untreated, toxicities may cause diminished quality of life and, at worst, mortality.

Whatever the healthcare setting, it is our role as healthcare professionals to encourage patients to discuss any side effects they may be experiencing as a result of cytotoxic treatment. This allows the assessment of toxicities to identify appropriate interventional strategies to mimimise the impact on health, as well as to support patients emotionally. The knowledge and experience you gain on your cancer/palliative care placement will be invaluable to help you do this on future placements and in practice.

References

Bergkvist, K., Wengstrom, Y., 2006. Symptom experiences during chemotherapy treatment – with focus on nausea and vomiting. European Journal of Oncology Nursing 10, 21–29.

Brown, M., 2010. Nursing care of patients undergoing allogeneic stem cell transplantation. Nursing Standard 25 (11), 47–56.

Coughlan, M., Healey, C., 2008. Nursing care, education and support for patients with neutropenia. Nursing Standard 22 (46), 35–41.

Irshad, S., Maisey, N., 2010. Considerations when choosing oral chemotherapy: identifying and responding to patient need. European Journal of Cancer Care (Engl.) 19, 5–11.

Methven, C., 2010. Effects of chemotherapy-induced neutropenia on quality of life. Cancer Nursing Practice 9 (1), 30–33.

Molassiotis, A., Stricker, C.T., Easby, B., et al., 2008. Understanding the concept of chemotherapy related nausea: the patient experience. European Journal of Cancer 17, 444–453.

Nikoletti, S., Hyde, S., Shaw, T., et al., 2005. Comparison of plain ice and flavoured ice for preventing oral mucositis associated with 5FU. Journal of Clinical Nursing 14 (6), 750–753.

Power, S., Condon, C., 2008. Chemotherapy-induced alopecia: a phenomenological study. Cancer Nursing Practice 7 (7), 44–47.

Raber-Durlacher, J.E., Elad, S., Barasch, A., 2010. Oral mucositis. Oral Oncology 46 (6), 452–456.

Van Achterberg, T., 2007. The effectiveness of commonly used mouthwashes for the prevention of chemotherapy-induced oral mucositis: a systematic review. European Journal of Cancer Care (Engl.) 15 (5), 431–439.

Van den Hurk, C.J., Mols, F., Vingerhoets, A.J., Breed, W.P., 2010. Impact of alopecia and scalp cooling on the well-being of breast cancer patients. Psychooncology 19 (7), 701–709.

Vento, S., Cainelli, F., 2003. Infections in patients with cancer undergoing chemotherapy: aetiology, prevention and treatment. Lancet 4 (10), 595–604.

Worthington, H.V., Clarkson, J.E., Bryan, G., et al., 2006. Interventions for preventing oral mucositis for patients with cancer receiving treatment. Cochrane Database Syst. Rev. doi:10.1002/14651858.CD000978. pub5.

Further reading

Baquiran, D.C., Gallagher, J., 2001. Cancer chemotherapy handbook, 2nd ed. Lippincott Williams and Wilkins, Baltimore.

Brighton, D., Wood, M., 2005. The Royal Marsden Hospital handbook of cancer chemotherapy. Churchill Livingstone, Edinburgh.

Coward, M., Coley, H.M., 2006. Chemotherapy. In: Kearney, N., Richardson, A. (Eds.), Nursing patients with cancer: principles and practice. Churchill Livingstone, Edinburgh.

Dougherty, L., Bailey, C., Chemotherapy. In: Corner, J., Bailey, C. (Eds.), Cancer nursing: care in context, 2nd ed. Blackwell, Oxford.

Duffy, L., 2009. Care of immunocompromised patients in hospital. Nursing Standard 23 (36), 35–41.

Maxwell, C.J., 2008. Putting evidence into practice: evidence-based interventions for the management of oral mucositis. Clinical Journal of Oncology Nursing 12 (1), 141–152.

Prescher-Hughes, D.S., Alkhoudairy, C.J., 2007. Clinical practice protocols in oncology nursing. Jones and Bartlett, Boston.

Yarbro, C.H., Hansen Frogge, M., Godman, M., 2004. Cancer symptom management. Jones and Bartlett, Boston.

Yarbro, C.H., Hansen Frogge, M., Godman, M., 2005. Cancer nursing: principles and practice, 6th ed. Jones and Bartlett, Boston.

Websites

European Oncology Nursing Society, http://www.cancernurse.eu/ (accessed May 2011).

Cancer Nursing education, videos and other learning materials, http://www.cancernursing.org/ (accessed May 2011).

Cancernausea.com Website (USA), http://www.cancernausea.com/.

Chemotherapy information, http://www.chemotherapy.com/ (accessed May 2011).

Charity Website with information and help with alopecia and wigs: http://www.mynewhair.org/Home.aspx (accessed May 2011).

National Institute for Health and Clinical Excellence, http://www.nice.org.uk/ (accessed May 2011).

NHS Choices, http://www.nhs.uk/Conditions/Chemotherapy/Pages/Definition.aspx (accessed May 2011).

Oncology Nursing Society (UK), http://www.ukons.org/ (accessed May 2011).

Oncology Nursing Society (USA), http://www.ons.org/ (accessed May 2011).

Royal College of Radiologists chemotherapy guidelines, http://www.rcr.ac.uk/ (accessed May 2011).

11 Caring for the patient undergoing haemopoietic stem cell transplant

CHAPTER AIMS

- To introduce the student to the principles of haemopoietic stem cell transplant
- To understand the impact of haemopoietic stem cell transplant on the individual
- To highlight the care required when nursing a patient undergoing haemopoietic stem cell transplant

Introduction

Patients with a haematological malignancy such as leukaemia, lymphoma and myeloma may undergo a haemopoietic stem cell transplant as part of their cancer treatment. This is a highly specialised procedure and is undertaken in a specialised transplant unit. If you have been allocated to a specialist transplant unit, you will have the opportunity to observe and experience high-intensity transplants and learn to care for acutely sick patients. If you have not been allocated to this area, you may be able to arrange an insight visit. Whether you get the opportunity to visit a haemopoietic transplant unit or not, you may meet individuals who are either preparing for the procedure or who have undergone the treatment. Increasingly, low-risk haemopoietic stem cell transplants are being performed in more general areas such as the community setting (Dix & Geller 2000). This requires community-based healthcare professionals to be knowledgeable and skilled in caring for these patients. Although the transplant phase is very intensive and patients can become critically unwell, patients require long-term support so you may meet these patients during the post-transplant phase.

Haemopoietic stem cell transplant is the use of high-dose cytotoxic therapy (with or without radiotherapy) and a transfusion of haemopoietic stem cells to 'rescue' the patient's haematological status. Previously, bone marrow was used in transplants, extracted from the iliac crest under local anaesthetic. This was painful and intrusive. To avoid this, stem cells are now used. Stem cells are the cells that develop into, or *differentiate* into, all types of blood cells – red and white cells and platelets – and can easily be accessed peripherally.

There are three types of haemopoietic transplant, depending on where the stems cells come from:

- *Autologous transplant*: this involves taking stems cells from the patient and then processing and freezing them.

The patient then receives high-dose cytotoxic therapy ± radiotherapy and this gets rid of the cancer cells. The frozen cells are defrosted and infused (like a blood transfusion) to repopulate the patient's bone marrow.

- *Syngeneic transplant*: this uses an identical twin's stem cells. This is essentially like an autologous transplant, but has a better chance of success.
- *Allogeneic transplant*: this uses stem cells from a donor (this may be a family member or a stranger on a national database) who has a similar *tissue type*. Either stem cells are removed from the peripheral blood, or umbilical cord blood may be used. When a baby is born, a mother can decide whether to have the umbilical cord blood frozen. This can be kept in case the child or a sibling requires a haemopoietic stem cell transplant in later life. Alternatively, it may be donated to the national database to be donated for an allogeneic transplant or it may be destroyed.

 Activity

Find out about how patients are matched to their donors. Think about what the ethical and psychological issues might be in receiving or donating stem cells. Should individuals conceive a baby in order to obtain umbilical cord blood for a sick child? What if no-one in the family is a match? What if the transplant does not work? How might the donor feel?

NMC Domain 1:1.1; 1.2
NMC Domain 2: 2.4
NMC Domain 3: 3.2

Whatever the type of haemopoietic transplant, the principles of treatment are similar. Before the stems cells can be collected, the number of peripheral stem cells must be increased – this is called *priming*. This can be achieved in two ways. First, subcutaneous (SC) injections of *colony-stimulating factors* (discussed in Ch. 12), such as *granulocyte colony-stimulating factor* (GCS-F) can be used. This growth factor stimulates the body's stem cells to divide and develop into more neutrophils. Second, cytotoxic therapy can be used. As the immune system recovers from being suppressed by the cytotoxic drugs, the number of stems cells in the peripheral blood increases. Eight to ten days after the cytotoxic drugs have been given, the stem cells can be harvested by a procedure called *apheresis*. This uses a machine called a cell separator which is attached to the patient via an intravenous cannula and only removes white blood cells. This process may take a few hours and may be performed several times until enough stem cells have been collected. The cells are then cryopreserved with a chemical and can be stored until required.

Once priming is complete, patients undergo *pretransplant conditioning*; this involves giving high-dose cytotoxic drugs. Sometimes *total body irradiation* (TBI) is also given. This serves two purposes: to reduce the number of cancer cells and to suppress the patient's immune system to prevent the rejection of the donor cells or graft. This will destroy bone marrow production and peripheral white blood cells, which would lead to death, so in order to rescue the immune system, the stored stem cells are transfused. Before the cells are infused, the patient receives IV fluids to hydrate them. The frozen cells are then defrosted gently and give intravenously. Patients may have an allergic reaction to the preserving chemical.

Side effects

Patients undergoing haemopoietic stem cell transplant experience similar side effects to patients receiving cytotoxics, however the toxicities are much more severe and last much longer. While the newly acquired stem cells establish themselves and replace the white blood cells, patients will have severe and prolonged neutropenia, making them highly susceptible to infection and sepsis. It is very common for patients to experience *anaemia* (low red blood cells) and *thrombocytopenia* (low platelets) (if all blood cells are reduced, this is called *pancytopenia*); veno-occlusive disease (small blood vessels in the liver become blocked); severe mucositis; nausea and vomiting; and diarrhoea.

Due to the severity of the risk of infection and other acute toxicities, patients are usually cared for in a single side room on a specialist transplant unit. Most patients become critically ill in the first few weeks and need very careful intensive nursing care.

The procedure is often associated with significant mortality and the physical and psychosocial status of patients is commonly disrupted and their recovery slow, affecting quality of life (Liptrott 2007).

Patients require frequent and regular haemodynamic monitoring (blood pressure; pulse; respirations; oxygen saturations; temperature; central venous pressure). They will need meticulous fluid balance monitoring and maintenance to ensure they are well hydrated and have good renal function; nutritional support (usually *total parenteral nutrition* (TPN) is given intravenously); oral care; personal hygiene; assessment and management of gastrointestinal disturbance (diarrhoea and nausea/vomiting); pain assessment; daily blood counts; and psychosocial assessment and support.

 Activity

Find out what types of pathogens commonly cause infections in immunosuppressed patients.

NMC Domain 3: 3.2

It usually takes a few weeks before it is known whether the transplant has been successful. If donor cells are used, there is a chance that the patient may reject the new stems cells. This is known as graft versus host disease (GVHD) and can cause debilitating side effects such as skin blistering, reduced liver function and gastrointestinal tract disturbance. There may be many severe long-term side effects of GVHD such as infertility, cataracts, reduced hormone production, pulmonary complications and relapse (Brown 2010). To minimise GVHD, immunosuppressive therapy is used, such as ciclosporin (given orally), which may be continued for months or years if the patient experiences chronic GVDH (Grundy 2006).

Having undergone a haemopoietic stem cell transplant, patients often experience long-term side effects that may be multidimensional, affecting the individual psychologically (loss of control; fear of relapse; facing own mortality; change of body image) as well the physically (loss of fertility; diminished physical strength and fatigue; secondary cancers).

Caring for patients

There has been a shift in how and where patients are cared for. More patients are receiving treatment at home following an autologous haemopoietic stem cell transplant. This means the patient receives their cytotoxic treatment as an inpatient and is then discharged home immediately to receive post-transplant care. Alternatively, they may receive their cytotoxic treatment and stem cell transplant at home under the care of a community-based haematology team. District nurses play an integral role in caring for these patients and will be involved in the care of central lines and the administration of antibiotics, as well as all aspects of care. This brings its own challenges as well as opportunities and improvements to the patient experience and outcome.

References

Brown, M., 2010. Nursing care of patients undergoing allogeneic stem cell transplantation. Nursing Standard 25 (11), 47–56.

Dix, S., Geller, R., 2000. High dose chemotherapy with autologous stem cell rescue in the outpatient setting. Oncology 14 (2), 171–186.

Grundy, M., 2006. Nursing in haematological oncology, 2nd ed. Baillière Tindall, Edinburgh.

Liptrott, S., 2007. Quality of life in stem cell transplant patients; a literature review. Cancer Nursing Practice 6 (10), 29–33.

Further reading

Ritchie, L., 2005. Outpatient stem cell transplant: effectiveness and implications. British Journal of Community Nursing 10 (1), 14.

Websites

American Cancer Society, http://www.cancer.org/Treatment/TreatmentsandSideEffects/TreatmentTypes/BoneMarrowandPeripheralBloodStemCellTransplant/index (accessed May 2011).

Leukaemia Society, http://www.leukaemiasociety.org/ (accessed May 2011).

Lymphoma Association, http://www.lymphomas.org.uk/info/treatments.asp (accessed May 2011).

Macmillan information for patients, http://www.macmillan.org.uk/Cancerinformation/Cancertreatment/Treatmenttypes/Stemcellbonemarrowtransplants/Highdosetreatment/Highdosetreatment.aspx (accessed May 2011).

Myeloma Association, http://www.myeloma.org.uk/ (accessed May 2011).

12

Caring for the patient undergoing biological therapy

CHAPTER AIM

- To introduce the principles of biological therapy
- To understand the impact of biological therapy on the individual

Introduction

One of the most exciting and most recent developments in cancer treatments are the biological therapies. These have been developed as a result of the expansion of our knowledge of cancer biology. Many of these treatments are still in the trial phase and are still being investigated to optimise their effectiveness and to identify what side effects they may cause. However NICE has approved many of these treatments for general use. During your cancer/palliative care placement, you may come across patients receiving biological therapies alongside other cancer treatments such as cytotoxic therapy or radiotherapy. If you are allocated to a cancer centre, you may be able to arrange an insight visit with the clinical research team who coordinate and run cancer clinical trials.

Many of the treatments are administered orally and patients who are physically able will self-administer the drugs at home, so you may encounter the treatments while on a community placement or in the outpatient setting. Alternatively, if you have a placement in an inpatient area, try to find out what biological treatments some of your patients are on. Patients often confuse these drugs with cytotoxic therapy, but they act very differently and the side effects of biological therapies are variable in terms of the range of toxicities as well as the severity.

Biological therapies are treatments that use natural substances from the body, or drugs made from these substances. Biological therapies stimulate, direct or boost the body's own immune cells to:

- attack or control the growth of cancer cells
- restore blood cells following an episode of cytotoxic-related neutropenia
- interfere with the way cells interact and signal to each other.

🕐 Activity

Read Waugh and Grant (2010) (see References) or a similar textbook to refresh your knowledge of the different parts and cells of the immune system. How does the immune system work to get rid of non-self cells?

NMC Domain 3: 3.2

Table 12.1 Types of biological therapies

Groups of biological therapies	Examples of agents
Cytokines	Interferon, interleukins, tumour necrosis factor, colony-stimulating factors (G-CSF: pegfilgrastim/filgrastim and epoetin alfa)
Monoclonal antibodies (MoAbs)	Trastuzumab (Herceptin), rituximab, bevacizumab, cetuximab
Cancer growth blockers	Tyrosine kinase inhibitors: erotinib (Tarceva), imatinib (Glivec), getitinib (Iressa), sunitinib, dasatinib, lapatinib Proteasome inhibitors: bortezomib (Velcade)
Anti-angiogenic agents	Thalidomide
Cancer vaccines	Bacillus Calmette–Guérin (BCG)
Gene therapies	In development

There are numerous types of biological therapies. Table 12.1 identifies some of the main groups and provides examples of drugs/agents. Each group is discussed in turn.

Cytokines

Cytokines are natural protein messengers secreted from blood cells that coordinate the immune system. They attach to a receptor on the surface of white blood cells and trigger them to multiply, recognise and deal with anything that is foreign to the body, such as a cancer cell, bacteria, etc.

Interferon is a cytokine that is produced when white blood cells come in contact with a virus. It interferes with the ability of the virus to reproduce and stops other cells becoming infected with the virus. Interferon alpha is given subcutaneously. It interferes with or stops the cancer's growth, makes cancer cells more vulnerable to being killed by white blood cells and reduces the number of blood vessels around the

cancer. Interferon alpha is used to treat renal cell cancers, melanoma and chronic myeloid leukaemia. It can also be given topically to treat some types of skin cancer.

Another group of cytokines are the interleukins which are given intravenously (Batchelor 2006).

Yet another group is the *haemopoietic growth factors*. These stimulate production of white blood cells and help them mature. Rather than being used to eliminate cancer, these factors can be made synthetically, and boost recovery of the immune system when it has been damaged by cytotoxic therapy. Generally, granulocyte colony-stimulating factor (G-CSF) is used subcutaneously to stimulate neutrophil production and maturation, to prevent or minimise the severity and length of neutropenia and to lower the risk of infection when a patient is undergoing cytotoxic therapy and is likely to become immunocompromised. G-CSF is also used in haemopoietic transplant to increase the number of stems cells in the blood, before harvesting (discussed in Ch. 11).

Monoclonal antibodies

All cells have growth factor receptors on their cell surface. These are known as *antigens.* Antigens are activated when they come in contact with a specific growth factor, which enables the cell to divide. Antigens are also used by the immune system to recognise non-self cells that might cause harm. When B lymphocytes come into contact with something unfamiliar like a cancer cell or bacteria, they make *B memory cells* that remember and recognise it more easily next time. The B cells also produce specific antibodies (proteins) in the plasma which lock on to the specific antigen to activate an *immune complex.* This then aids other white cells to *phagocytose* (engulf) and destroy the foreign cell.

Some cancer cells have too many antigens on the surface which signal for increased cell division. To stop the cancer cells dividing, more copies of the specific antibody can be manufactured in the form of monoclonal antibodies (MoAbs). MoAbs inhibit cancer cellular growth by blocking the specific growth factor that tells the cell to divide. They also make these cancer cells more recognisable, so the white cells can kill them. For example, normal cells have two copies of human epidermal growth factor 2 (HER2) receptor protein. These cell receptors lock together with growth factors and trigger the cell to grow. Approximately 30–40% of patients with breast cancer have too many HER2 receptors as a result of an amplification of a gene which increases cell division. A MoAb known as *trastuzumab* (Herceptin) can be given intravenously and will attach to the receptors, blocking growth, slowing cell division and contributing to cell death. MoAbs are often given with cytotoxic drugs to increase the effectiveness of treatment. Other MoAbs include rituximab used to treat non-Hodgkin's lymphoma, bevacizumab (Avastin) and cetuximab

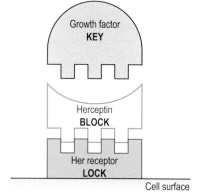

Fig 12.1 MoAb: Herceptin blocking cell surface receptor HER2

used to control metastatic colorectal and breast cancer.

Not all patients (even with cancer cells with extra receptors) will respond. Cancer cells can learn to avoid binding to the antibodies, by downregulating (reducing) the number of receptors available. In addition, MoAbs are big molecules and cannot reach all the cells in a large cancer which has narrow blood vessels (Fig. 12.1).

Cancer growth blockers

Growth factors tell the cell when to divide, when to stop dividing and when to become specialised. They do this by attaching to a receptor on the cell surface, which sends a signal inside the cell which then sets off a number of reactions. All growth factors work with each other and each growth factor has a specific receptor. An example of this is epidermal growth factor (EGF): it attaches itself to epidermal growth factor receptors (EGFRs) on the cell surface and activates an enzyme called *tyrosine kinase*, which in turn triggers the cancer cell to divide. One group of cancer growth blockers are the tyrosine kinase inhibitors (TKIs). Erotinib (Tarveva) is a TKI, given orally, used to treat non-small cell lung cancer. Erotinib targets the inside part of the EGFR and prevents tyrosine kinase being activiated, thus stopping the cell from dividing.

Another group of cancer growth blockers are the proteasome inhibitors. Proteasomes help break down proteins (that are not required) into small pieces so the cell can reuse them. If proteasomes are blocked, the proteins will build up and the cell will die. Bortezomib (Velcade) is a proteasome inhibitor used to treat myeloma.

Other agents

Other biological therapies include anti-angiogenic agents such as thalidomide. Used in the 1960s to treat nausea in pregnancy, thalidomide was found to suppress the formation of blood vessels which is essential for cancer to spread. It has been used with relative success in patients with myeloma.

Cancer vaccines are being developed that involve injection of a weak strain of a cancer antigen. The B cells recognise it and produce specific antibodies that then lock onto many of the cancer antigens, allowing the immune system to recognise and kill the cancer cells.

Another vaccine, Bacillus Calmette–Guérin (BCG) was develop to treat tuberculosis, but has been used to treat superficial bladder cancer, by causing a local immune reaction.

Based on the fundamental basis that cancer is a genetic disease, caused by an accumulation of mutations in the DNA, gene therapy is an important development in which a new, undamaged gene could be introduced into a patient to replace the damaged gene. The new gene could correct the cellular processes and control cell division. The downside to this is that a cancer results from many genetic errors and each of these would need to be replaced.

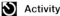 **Activity**

Identify a patient undergoing a biological cancer treatment. Find out what type of biological therapy they are receiving and the side effects they have experienced.

NMC Domain 1: 1.4
NMC Domain 2: 2.3
NMC Domain 3: 3.1; 3.3; 3.6; 3.7

Side effects of biological therapies

Because biological therapies are boosting the body's own immune system to kill cancer cells, normal cells are not damaged in the process. This means that the range of side effects is much narrower than with other treatments. The side effects are generally a result of an immune response: hypersensitivity, flu-like symptoms, fever, rigors, muscle/joint pain, nausea, skin reaction, hypotension, diarrhoea and fatigue. Herceptin may cause long-term cardiac toxicities, especially combined with anthracycline cytotoxic drugs, although the full impact of this is not yet known.

Whatever clinical environment you are working in, you are likely to meet patients undergoing biological therapy as these treatments are becoming increasingly important to control and remove cancer cells.

References

Batchelor, D., 2006. Biological therapy. In: Kearney, N., Richardson, A. (Eds.), Nursing patients with cancer: principles and practice. Churchill Livingstone, Edinburgh.

Waugh, A., Grant, A., 2010. Ross and Wilson anatomy and physiology in health and illness. Churchill Livingstone, Edinburgh.

Further reading

Battiato, L.A., 2005. Biological and targeted therapy. In: Yarbro, C.H., Hansen Frogge, M., Godman, M. (Eds.), Cancer nursing: principles and practice. sixth ed. Jones and Bartlett, Boston.

Pecorino, L., 2008. Molecular biology of cancer: mechanisms, targets and therapeutics, second ed. Oxford University Press, Oxford.

Souhami, R., Tobias, J., 2005. Cancer and its management, fifth ed. Blackwell, Oxford.

Yarbro, C.H., Hansen Frogge, M., Godman, M., 2004. Cancer symptom management. Jones and Bartlett, Boston.

13 Caring for the patient undergoing radiotherapy

CHAPTER AIMS

- To introduce the principles of radiotherapy
- To understand the impact of radiotherapy on the individual
- To highlight the care required when nursing a patient undergoing radiotherapy

Introduction

Radiotherapy has been a key treatment for cancer for over a century and although the fundamental principles of treatment have not changed, the method of delivery and the treatment techniques have changed considerably. Most patients diagnosed with cancer undergoing radiotherapy will receive their treatment as an outpatient, so you may meet them in the community setting or in an outpatient unit, or on a ward if they are admitted for a treatment-related problem or other medical condition. Radiotherapy remains misunderstood by patients and it is often feared due to association with radiation disasters and misuse. It is important while on a cancer/palliative placement that you make the most of the opportunity to understand this treatment; arrange an insight visit to the radiotherapy department to observe the equipment and to understand the complexity of planning radiotherapy and to appreciate the experience of patients.

After surgery, radiotherapy is the most effective curative treatment for cancer (Burnet et al 2000). Approximately 50% of patients in the UK will receive radiotherapy. Unlike the treatments discussed in previous chapters that are given systemically, the value of radiotherapy is in the local management of cancer. The success of radiotherapy is dependent on how bulky the tumour is, how sensitive the tissues are to radiation and the location of the tumour.

Radiation is a natural part of the electromagnetic spectrum. At one end of the electromagnetic spectrum are radio waves which have low energy and bounce around us; at the other end of the spectrum, X-rays, beta and gamma rays are highly energised and can penetrate into the body, causing *ionisation*. Ionisation is where the atoms within the cell are altered by the radiation. Atoms are electrical in nature. When they come into contact with radiation, the highly energised waves from the radiation cause an orbiting electron to be dislodged and join an adjacent atom which is said to be ionised (Fig. 13.1).

Whether an atom has lost or gained an electron, the atom becomes unstable and the cell DNA becomes damaged (especially

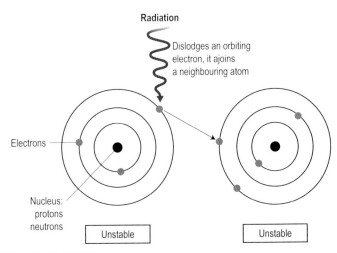

Fig 13.1 Ionisation of atoms

when the cell is dividing), causing the cell to die. Similar to cytotoxic drugs, radiotherapy will damage and kill healthy cells as well as cancer cells. Normal cells have the ability to repair and replace themselves when they are damaged though.

X-rays, beta and gamma rays have the right amount of energy to produce ionisation in atoms, which takes place as radiation passes through tissue. Different tissues have different levels of sensitivity to radiation. This will affect the success of the treatment but also restricts the dose that can be given.

Radiotherapy is measured in Grays (Gy), the amount of radiation absorbed by tissues (1 Gy = 1 joule of energy absorbed per Kg of tissue). Cancers that are radio-sensitive (lymphomas, germ cell cancers) are given lower doses (20–45 Gy), while those that are radio-resistant (gliomas, prostate, adenocarcinomas) are given higher doses (60–70 Gy).

External beam radiation is the commonest type of radiation treatment.

It is given in the outpatient setting using beams of radiation that are artificially made by accelerating X-rays using a machine called a *linear accelerator* (Linac).

There are four principles ('four Rs') that support our understanding of how radiotherapy works:
- Repair: radiotherapy damages cells both directly and indirectly. Directly, if the damage to DNA is great, the repair genes will not be able to fix the problem and the cell will commit suicide or undergo apoptosis. Indirectly, the radiotherapy interacts with oxygen and water molecules in the cell to damage DNA as it is synthesised. Very few cells are killed straight away – it takes several cell divisions before the cell dies. Cells that die immediately are very radiosensitive, such as lymphocytes and germ cells. These are very vulnerable and responsive to radiotherapy.
- Reoxygenation: the success of radiotherapy depends on the presence of oxygen. Many cancers have a poor

blood supply and are often hypoxic. This reduces the indirect action of radiotherapy which requires oxygen to damage the synthesis of DNA. To maximise the amount of oxygen, external radiotherapy is generally given in fractions. These are individual doses of radiotherapy which allow well-oxygenated cells to be killed, making way for hypoxic cells to have access to more oxygen, making them more sensitive to the next fraction of radiotherapy. Fractionisation also allows normal cells to repair and repopulate which minimises side effects.

- Redistribution: those cells in G0 will not be killed initially as they are not actively in the cell cycle, but as cells that are actively cycling die, cells in G0 are recruited into the cell cycle to replace damaged cells. Giving fractions over a period of days/weeks means that cells are more likely to be in the cell cycle and be killed. Cells are most sensitive in the M and G2 phase.
- Repopulation: cancer cells that are not actively dividing when the radiotherapy is given will start to divide after the dose, in order to replace those cells destroyed. If another dose of radiation is given, these cells will also be damaged. If the cancer repopulation happens more quickly than the radiotherapy is given, the success of the treatment will be reduced. For example, when radiotherapy is given, a number of cancer cells are killed off and other cancer cells repopulate to replace those lost. If there is a delay in the treatment schedule, these cancer cells will continue replicating, reducing the chance of success. Some radiotherapy schedules, such as accelerated hyperfractionated (CHART) radiotherapy, are give twice a day to try to deal with the problem of cancer cells repopulating more quickly than normal cells.

Careful planning of radiotherapy is essential to maximise the effects and minimise the damage to sensitive surrounding tissues and this may take time and delay treatment. X-rays and magnetic resonance imaging (MRI) scans are used to identify the location of the cancer. These scans are loaded into a planning computer to ascertain the shape and size of the treatment field. To minimise the damage to sensitive structures and tissues, the smallest area possible is treated. Shields and moulds are used to shape the beams and control the depth of penetration. A mask may be made if an area of the body needs to be immobilised to ensure precision, such as the head and neck. The dose and number of fractions are calculated and a machine called a simulator (a diagnostic X-ray machine) is used to give a dry run to check the accuracy and to make any adjustments. The information from the simulator is then used by the radiographer to deliver the radiotherapy exactly as planned.

Activity

Visit the radiotherapy department and watch how a mask for head and neck radiotherapy is made. Find out how a patient's radiotherapy is planned using the simulator. Escort a patient to radiotherapy. Find out about how the patient is positioned and how the machine is set up. If you are in a clinical area where this does not happen, discuss with your mentor about arranging a spoke placement or an insight visit to observe radiotherapy being planned and given.

NMC Domain 3: 3.1; 3.2; 3.4; 3.6

Seeing this for yourself will help you to reassure patients who are undergoing radiotherapy that you might meet while on another placement.

External beam radiotherapy is particularly good in the management of symptoms. Because of the way radiation works, the cells do not immediately die and the treatment may initially cause exacerbation of symptoms, which may increase distress and anxiety. Many patients experience bone pain (often caused by bone metastases). Bone pain is often unresponsive to pharmaceutical drugs but generally is responsive to radiotherapy. Radiotherapy to the site(s) of the cancer in the bone will kill the cancer cells and stimulate new bone growth. It takes several days, and up to 2 weeks before the full benefit is achieved and pain is reduced. During this time, the level of analgesia should be maintained and the patient should be informed that there will be a delayed response.

 Activity

> Read Rosenfield and Stahl (2006) (see References). Discuss the role of radiotherapy and the use of other strategies used to manage bone pain, and the nursing implications for each, with your mentor
>
> NMC Domain 3: 3.1; 3.2; 3.4; 3.6

Nerve and visceral pain can also be difficult to manage as the cancer invades, compresses and distorts organs. Radiotherapy reduces the size of the cancer and relieves pressure and inflammation.

Hepatic pain is very sensitive to radiotherapy which can relieve jaundice by reducing hepatobiliary obstruction.

Brain metastases respond well to radiotherapy and 80% of patients with cerebral metastases experience symptomatic relief, with a reduction in headaches, seizures and blurred vision. Again, it takes time for the treatment to work and the average response time is 10 weeks. This has obvious implications for patients with a short life expectancy. Patients often require hospitalisation during or post-treatment

due to increased symptoms initially, such as seizures, headaches, increased cranial pressure, etc. The use of steroids can help alleviate this exacerbation of symptoms.

Bleeding such as haemoptysis, fistulas, ulcerated and fungating wounds (caused by cancer breaking through the skin) can also be managed by radiotherapy, to reduce discomfort and stem bleeding. In addition, improvements can be achieved in breathlessness and dysphagia. Spinal cord compression requires urgent radiotherapy to reduce the pressure on the spinal cord. By killing the cancer cells and allowing bone reformation, *some* motor function may be regained. This is dependent on the degree of damage caused initially.

Where radiotherapy is used to palliatiate symptoms rather than as a definitive treatment, the effects will only last until the cancer grows. This condition is explained more fully in Chapter 15.

Other radiation treatments

Radiation can also be used directly inside the body. These treatments are referred to as brachytherapy (sealed) and unsealed sources. Caesium 137, a sealed radioactive isotope, can be placed inside the body. This is often used for gynaecological cancers like endometrial or cervical cancer. Usually the patient will have surgery and a course of external beam radiotherapy and will then be admitted for the internal radiation. A set of applicators (either two or three) are inserted vaginally and packed into place under a general anaesthetic and a urinary catheter is inserted. The patient will then have their treatment planned using the simulator (mentioned above). They are then returned to the ward and placed in a lead-lined room. The applicators are connected to tubes that are attached to a machine known as a *selectron*. When the machine is switched on, radioactive caesium pellets travel down the tubes and into the applicators inside the patient. These pellets deliver radiation directly to the area where the cancer is. The patient is nursed flat and must not move in case of dislodging the applicators. They will require postoperative care and regular pain management. As and when the patient needs assistance, the selectron machine can be turned off and the radioactive pellets returned into a safe. This means it is safe for nurses to attend to the patient without coming into contact with the radiation. Up until recently, patients received their selectron treatment as an inpatient and were attached to the machine for between 10 and 20 hours, however an increasing number of cancer centres have introduced this treatment as a day case. The procedure, known as low-dose rate selectron, is similar to the inpatient treatment, but the patient receives a short anaesthetic, the applicators are left in place and the patient will receive treatment over a few days as a day case.

An example of a sealed radioactive treatment is *iridium wires* which are inserted into the skin and tissues under a general anaesthetic. These wires are used to treat anal, vaginal and urethral cancers. The risk to healthcare professionals is much higher with this treatment as the radiation cannot be temporarily removed and the patient will be radioactive for the duration of the treatment. Similarly, *iodine 131* is an unsealed source which is given as an oral capsule or liquid. When consumed it is absorbed into the thyroid gland and cancer cells in the thyroid will be killed. This is used in conjunction with, or instead of, a thyroidectomy. Because the iodine 131 is given orally, these patients will stay radioactive until the radiation starts to degrade – this may be several weeks. Patients who have had iodine 131 are required to stay in a lead-lined room for between 4 and 7 days (depending on the time taken to degrade the radioactivity). During their admission, patients are highly radioactive, therefore they should require minimal assistance with their activities of daily living and self-administer their medications, minimising contact with healthcare professionals. As a student, you should not enter a patient's room if they have received either iodine 131 or iridium wires. This is discussed in Chapter 7 under health and safety issues.

While undergoing iodine 131 treatment, the patient will only be allowed to use disposable crockery and cutlery. All surfaces are covered in a plastic film to minimise radiation contamination from the patient's sweat and the medical team will closely monitor the radiation levels.

It can be very lonely being isolated for such a time, therefore patients should be advised to bring plenty of activities such as books, puzzles, DVDs, music, games, laptops, etc. However, they need to be aware that everything they bring in with them will be monitored for radioactivity. If the levels of radiation in the patient's belongings are not at a safe level at the time of discharge, the items are retained by the hospital and placed in the radiotherapy 'bunker' (essentially a lead-lined store room) until the radiation has degraded, at which time they are returned to the patient. The patient will also be radioactive on discharge. Although the radioactive levels will have reduced to a safe level for them to return home, as a precaution they should avoid contact with children and pregnant women. They should use separate crockery and cutlery and sleep in a different room to their partner for a few weeks after treatment.

Activity

Read Stajduhar et al (2000) (see References). Think about the preparation, care and safety issues that are required in delivering this treatment.

NMC Domain 3: 3.1; 3.3; 3.4; 3.6

The impact of undergoing radiotherapy

Patients often are frightened or misunderstand what radiotherapy treatment actually is. This is often based on catastrophic events such as the World War Two atomic bombings of the Japanese cities of Nagasaki and Hiroshima and the nuclear power disasters in Chernobyl in the Ukraine in 1986 and Japan in 2011. Because of the technical nature of the treatment, patients and healthcare professionals often lack knowledge and understanding of how radiotherapy works. It is an abstract concept compared to surgical treatment where the cancer is physically removed or cytotoxic drugs are seen to enter the body. Radiotherapy is invisible. Peck and Boland (1977) demonstrated that approximately 60% of patients feel unprepared for treatment. Although this research is old, the figure is still relevant today. Information is required to outline what is involved in radiotherapy planning; how the treatment works; what to expect while in the radiotherapy department; the practicalities, such as parking; the duration of each treatment; what the likely side effects are and how these can be prevented; who to tell if a toxicity develops, etc. (Halkett et al 2010).

Because of the location of cancer centres with a radiotherapy department, patients might be required to travel long distances or they may be required to stay overnight.

The side effects of radiotherapy are varied and depend on the site of treatment. Severe toxicities may limit the dose that can be given, prolonging treatment time and the overall efficacy of treatment. However, the frequency and severity of radiotherapy side effects has reduced significantly due to developments in planning and delivery.

Like cytotoxic therapy, radiotherapy kills cells that are frequently dividing, so any normal cell that is active in the cell cycle and comes in contact with the radiation will potentially be damaged or killed. As all external radiotherapy beams have to enter the body through the skin, adverse skin reactions are common. The severity of the damage will depend on the dose; the number of fractions; and site of treatment (skin folds and areas of friction are more likely to increase the risk of a skin reaction). Exposure to sunlight will increase the risk of damage as will mechanical irritation such as clothes rubbing, shaving, etc. (Porock et al 2004). Other factors will influence how quickly and easily the body repairs the damage to the skin, such as age (the older we get, the slower the body repairs damage) and increased body weight (reduces healing, reduces blood supply, increased skin folds, friction and moisture).

Skin radiation reactions are often called 'radiation burns'. This is incorrect as the reaction is a repeated insult and is very different in nature to a normal burn.

To minimise radiation skin reaction, patients should be advised to wash their skin gently with mild soap and warm water; shaving the area of treatment should be avoided and clothing should be made from natural fibres that do not rub. When assisting a patient undergoing radiotherapy with their hygiene needs in an inpatient setting, you should also follow this advice. Patients should have their skin assessed throughout and after treatment to identify reaction and for prompt intervention (NHS Quality Improvement Scotland 2004). Eighty per cent of patients undergoing radiotherapy experience *erythema*, a redness and slight inflammation of the site, which occurs approximately 10–14 days after the first fraction. This coincides with the damaged basal layers migrating to the upper layers of the skin. The skin compensates by increasing cell division to replace the damaged cells. The new cells are immature and are more easily damaged. If the new cells are produced quicker than the old ones are shed, then *dry desquamation* develops;

this looks like dry, flaky, itchy skin. If the old cells are shed before the new ones can reach the top, then the thin epidermal layer is easily eroded; this is known as *moist desquamation*. Moist desquamation is more likely to develop in skin folds like under the breast, groin and axilla. When the skin breaks down, there is a high infection risk and the wound must be managed carefully to avoid further damage so that healing is promoted (MacBride et al 2008).

Another commonly reported general side effect is extreme fatigue. This tends to increase over the period of treatment. It is estimated that between 30% and 80% of patients undergoing radiotherapy will experience fatigue. This range is so wide, reflecting the subjective nature of the symptom and the difficulty in measuring fatigue (Jereczek-Fossa et al 2002). It is not clear why radiotherapy causes fatigue. It may be caused by travelling to and from the hospital daily and other side effects like loss of sleep, and the effort of the continual renewal of damaged cells. As well as the general side effects, there are usually a number of site-specific toxicities depending on the site of the radiotherapy (Table 13.1).

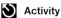 **Activity**

Read Hollinworth and Mann (2010) (see References) and find out how radiation skin reactions are treated in your area. Which dressings are used? How are dressings held in place? What can be done to promote wound healing in a radiotherapy-related wound?

NMC Domain 3: 3.1; 3.2; 3.3; 3.4; 3.6

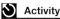 **Activity**

What advice could be given to a patient to help minimise fatigue while they undergo radiotherapy? Find out if a fatigue assessment tool is used in your area. Find out what strategies patients might use to manage the effects of fatigue.

NMC Domain 1: 1.4
NMC Domain 2: 2.6
NMC Domain 3: 3.1; 3.2; 3.3; 3.4; 3.7; 3.9; 3.10

Table 13.1 Site-specific radiotherapy side effects

Site of radiotherapy	Specific toxicities
Chest	Cough, oesophagitis, pain, pneumonitis, lung fibrosis, spinal cord damage, dyspnoea, nausea, indigestion
Breast (may include the axilla)	Mild breast oedema, lymphoedema in arm, brachial plexopathy, pain, breast shrinkage, lung fibrosis, bone necrosis (ribs), cardiac damage
Brain	Cerebral oedema (may cause raised intercranial pressure), alopecia, exacerbation of existing symptoms, somnolence (sleeping), white matter changes, cognitive changes, reduced hormone production

Continued

Table 13.1 Site-specific radiotherapy side effects—cont'd

Site of radiotherapy	Specific toxicities
Abdomen/pelvis	Abdominal cramps, diarrhoea, proctitis (inflammation of the anus and rectum), tenesmus (feeling of incomplete defecation) discharge, cystitis, frequency and urgency, incontinence, dysuria, infection, bowel and/or vaginal stenosis, fistula, impotence, infertility
Head and neck	Mucositis, infection, dysphagia, taste alteration, weight loss, increased salivary production (late effects might be reduced saliva production), dental caries, trismus (lock jaw), bone necrosis

The side effects of radiotherapy take a while to develop but last for a long time, often months after the completion of treatment. This is due to the indirect action of the treatment. The side effects may be temporary or permanent – either way, the majority of patients' functioning and quality of life are affected in some way. Knowing what toxicities to expect is important in order for prompt intervention. However, patients may not recognise the cause of the symptom they are experiencing and others are reluctant to report problems, in fear that treatment may be reduced or withdrawn.

References

Burnet, N., Benson, R., Williams, M., 2000. Improving cancer outcomes through radiotherapy. British Medical Journal 320, 198–199.

Halkett, G., Kristjanson, L., Lobb, E., 2010. Meeting breast cancer patients' information needs during radiotherapy: what can we do to improve the information and support that is currently provided? European Journal of Cancer Care (Engl.) 19 (4), 538–547.

Hollinworth, H., Mann, L., 2010. Managing acute skin reactions to radiotherapy treatment. Nursing Standard 24 (24), 53–54.

Jereczek-Fossa, B.A., Marsiglia, H.R., Orecchia, R., 2002. Radiotherapy-related fatigue. Critical Reviews in Oncology/Hematology 41, 317–325.

MacBride, S., Wells, M., Hornsby, C., et al., 2008. A case study to evaluate a new soft silicone dressing, Mepilex Lite, for patients with radiation skin reactions. Cancer Nursing 31 (1), E8–E14.

NHS Quality Improvement Scotland, 2004. Skincare of patients receiving radiotherapy: best practice statement. NHS Quality Improvement Scotland, Edinburgh.

Peck, A., Boland, J., 1977. Emotional reactions to radiation treatment. Cancer 40, 180–184.

Porock, D., Nikoletti, S., Cameron, F., 2004. The relationship between factors that impair wound healing and the severity of acute radiation skin and mucosal toxicities in head and neck. Cancer Nursing 27 (1), 1–78.

Rosenfield, R., Stahl, D., 2006. Pain management of bone metastases in breast cancer. Journal of Hospice and Palliative Nursing 8 (4), 233.

Stajduhar, K., Neithercut, J., Chu, E., 2000. Thyroid cancer: patients' experiences of receiving iodine-131 therapy. Oncology Nursing Forum 27 (8), 1213.

Further reading

Bolderston, A., 2006. The prevention and management of acute skin reactions related to radiation therapy: a systematic review and practice guideline. Support. Care Cancer 14 (8), 802–817.

Faithfull, S., 2006. Radiotherapy. In: Kearney, N., Richardson, A. (Eds.), Nursing patients with cancer: principles and practice. Churchill Livingstone, Edinburgh.

Faithfull, S., 2008. Radiotherapy. In: Corner, J., Bailey, C. (Eds.), Cancer nursing: care in context. 2nd ed. Blackwell, Oxford.

Faithfull, S., Wells, M., 2003. Supportive care in radiotherapy. Churchill Livingstone, Edinburgh.

Porock, D., 2002. Factors influencing the severity of radiation skin and oral mucosal reactions: development of a conceptual framework. European Journal of Cancer Care (Engl.) 11, 33–43.

Souhami, R., Tobias, J., 2005. Cancer and its management, 5th ed. Blackwell, Oxford.

Yarbro, C.H., Hansen Frogge, M., Godman, M., 2004. Cancer symptom management. Jones and Bartlett, Boston.

Yarbro, C.H., Hansen Frogge, M., Godman, 2005. Cancer nursing: principles and practice, 6th ed. Jones and Bartlett, Boston.

Websites

NHS Choices, http://www.nhs.uk/conditions/radiotherapy/Pages/Introduction.aspx (accessed May 2011).

Royal College of Radiologists, http://www.rcr.ac.uk/ (accessed May 2011).

14 Caring for the patient undergoing endocrine therapy

CHAPTER AIMS

- To introduce the principles of endocrine therapy
- To understand the impact of endocrine therapy on the individual
- To highlight the care required when nursing a patient undergoing endocrine therapy

Introduction

Many patients with hormone-responsive cancer receive endocrine therapy as part of their treatment, often as an adjuvant after surgery, cytotoxic therapy and radiotherapy. However, this treatment often has a lower profile than many of the other therapies and the side effects of endocrine therapy are often overlooked by healthcare professionals and under-reported by patients. One of the reasons for this is because patients receive endocrine therapy as outpatients and have less contact with healthcare professionals. In addition, the toxicities can be ambiguous and patients often don't know whether they should report the side effect or who they should tell and they are often embarrassed due to the nature of the side effects.

You may meet patients undergoing endocrine therapy in many healthcare settings, whether in the community or an inpatient ward or even a non-cancer placement, as patients may have been taking endocrine therapy for a number of years and may be admitted for another, non-cancer-related reason during that time. It is therefore important that you understand how the treatment works and how patients might be affected in order to provide support and information.

In Chapter 2, we discussed how some cancer cells grow in the presence of hormones (chemical messengers). Using this knowledge, endocrine or hormone therapy is a way of manipulating a patient's hormones to reduce the growth of a cancer or prevent it from growing back.

Activity

Read Waugh and Grant (2010) (see References) or a similar textbook and make a list of the tissues/organs that are under the control of hormones. What is the role of these hormones and how might they influence cancer growth?

NMC Domain 3: 3.2

Hormones are specific, targeting certain cells in order to act, controlling growth and maturation of organs. The hypothalamus gland is the master, controlling which hormones are produced. It produces a number of *hormone releasing hormones* that trigger the pituitary gland to release a range of hormones that target certain organs in the body that then produce the hormone end product.

To give an example, the hypothamus produces luteinising hormone-releasing hormone (LHRH), which in turn stimulates the pituitary to release luteinising hormone, which stimulates the ovary to produce oestrogen which then triggers ovulation. Figure 14.1 identifies the hormone pathways particularly significant in cancer.

Hormone levels are controlled by a process of *negative feedback*: in a situation where there is too much hormone, there is a signal to the hypothalamus and/or pituitary which inhibits and reduces the hormone production; where there is not enough hormone, a signal to the hypothalamus and/or pituitary increases production. Another way of controlling hormone levels is by increasing the numbers of cell receptors on the cell surface. If there is too much hormone, the number of cell receptors decreases – *downregulation* – and where there is too little, the number increases – *upregulation*.

How endocrine treatments work

Cancers that arise from organs normally under hormonal control may be treated by endocrine therapy, namely breast, prostate, thyroid and endometrial cancers. Endocrine therapy either blocks hormones, increases hormones or inhibits the conversion of hormones. Generally, these treatments are not curative, but are useful neoadjuvantly, adjuvantly, palliatively and possibly as a preventative measure. Sometimes endocrine therapy is used as a sole treatment, where other treatments such as surgery are not

recommended or a patient wishes to undergo a less invasive treatment. One of the reasons why endocrine therapy does not get rid of cancer completely is because as the cancer mutates, the cells look and behave differently to one another. Often some of the cells will be responsive to endocrine treatment, while others will not be. Sometimes a cancer will respond initially, but may become less responsive as the cancer mutates further. As stated in Chapter 2, at diagnosis a patient is tested to see if the cancer is sensitive to hormones. Sixty-five per cent of women with breast cancer will be oestrogen positive – these tend to be older women and they are more likely to have a better prognosis.

Tamoxifen is probably one of the oldest endocrine therapies. It enters the target cell and binds to a receptor, preventing the normal reaction taking place and slowing/stoping cell division. Fulvestrant works in a similar way by blocking the receptor; it also downregulates the number of cell surface receptors, making the cell less sensitive to the hormone. This drug may be used if a patient is resistant to tamoxifen. Goserelin (Zoladex) is an LHRH given as a subcutaneous injection. Once in the body, the LHRH stimulates the production of luteinising hormone and ultimately oestrogen. This surge of oestrogen triggers the negative feedback and stops production of oestrogen for a number of weeks. This drug is commonly used in premenopausal women. Goserelin has recently been trialled in women with breast cancer having cytotoxic drugs, to stop ovulation in an attempt to preserve fertility.

Remember that oestrogen is not only produced by the ovaries but also by the adipose tissues. After the menopause, a woman will continue to produce oestrogen because aromatase enzymes convert androgens into oestrogen. To stop this, the *aromatase inhibitors* (such as anastrozole) bind with the enzyme and stop the

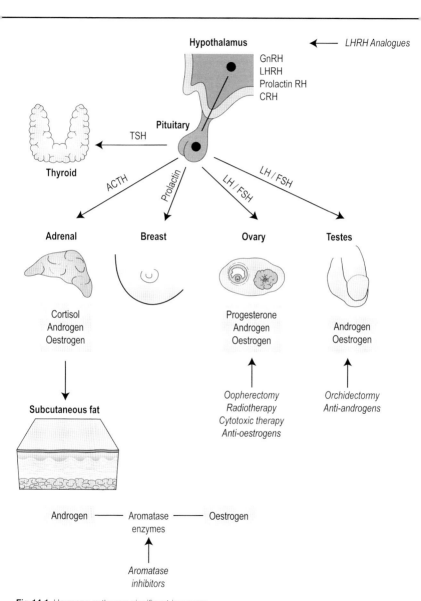

Fig 14.1 Hormone pathways significant in cancer

Table 14.1 Types of endocrine drugs

Type of cancer	Type of endocrine therapy	Examples of agents
Breast cancer (pre- and postmenopausal)	Selective oestrogen receptor modulator (SERM)	Tamoxifen, droloxifene, idoxifene, raloxifene
Breast cancer (postmenopausal)	Aromatase inhibitors	Anastrozole, letrozole, exemestane
Breast cancer (postmenopausal)	Selective oestrogen receptor downregulator	Fulvestrant
Breast cancer (premenopausal)	LHRH analogues	Goserelin (Zoladex)
Endometrial cancer Prostate cancer (rarely)	Additive hormonal therapies	Megestrol acetate (Megace) and medroxyprogesterone (Provera)
Prostate cancer	LHRH analogues	Goserelin (Zoladex)
Prostate cancer	Anti-androgens	Steroidal: cyproterone acetate (Cyprostat) Non-steroidal: (flutamide TDS, nilutamide, bicalutamide/casodex)
Prostate cancer	Oestrogens	Stilboestrol

conversion. These drugs are now recommended by NICE (2006) for postmenopausal women with primary breast disease.

Patients with prostate cancer generally respond well to endocrine therapy. Luteinising hormone-releasing hormone (LHRH) analogues are given adjuvantly after surgery; anti-androgens are often combined and used neoadjuvantly or as a sole treatment. Oestrogens are not used as much for prostate cancer as their side effects are severe and unpleasant.

Table 14.1 summarises the main endocrine therapies

Other ways of manipulating hormones is surgically (oophorectomy or orchidectomy) or by giving radiation to the ovaries or testes. This is a drastic action as it is permanent and, with the development of the drug therapies, is rarely done. Oestrogen production can also be reduced by using cytotoxic drugs, although this is not the primary aim of chemotherapy. A woman may experience an early menopause, especially if in their late 40s.

Side effects

Many of the endocrine therapies have undesirable effects causing physical discomfort and psychological trauma. The side effects are often under-reported and undiagnosed as the patient has been discharged from hospital and the effects develop gradually and can become chronic. Some of the common toxicities include the following:

- Hot flushes and sweating.
- Nausea and vomiting.

- Weight gain (commonly weight increase around abdomen and more likely if combined with chemotherapy (Goodwin et al 1999)).
- Vaginal bleeding and discharge.
- Thromboembolic disease (deep vein thrombosis (DVT)/pulmonary embolism (PE)).
- Visual disturbances.
- Modest increased risk of endometrial cancer.
- Joint stiffness and bone pain; hair thinning mild/moderate.
- Fatigue.
- Insomnia.
- Headaches.
- Bone mineral density disturbance and increased plasma lipids with the aromatase inhibitors.

Activity

Identify a patient undergoing endocrine therapy. Ask what side effects they have experienced. Then look up the drug. What are the common side effects caused by this drug specifically? Does the patient's experience reflect the expected side effects? How are the patient's physical functioning, psychological and social status affected? If you do not encounter a patient receiving endocrine therapy while on placement, look up a few of the drugs identified in Table 14.1. Make a few notes on how the drug is administered and what the common side effects are. This information can be useful to help you prepare for patient care.

NMC Domain 3: 3.1; 3.2; 3.3; 3.4; 3.6; 3.7; 3.8

Men often experience erectile dysfunction and develop female physical characteristics such as higher pitched voice, breast enlargement and hot sweats. This can be quite distressing and can influence an individual's sexuality and body image.

Because goserelin (Zoladex) creates a surge in hormone, patients may experience *tumour flare*, which may temporarily increase pain and hypercalcaemia (if they have bone metastases). Patients need to be aware of this before receiving treatment as the increase in pain can cause considerable physical distress, requiring additional analgesia, as well as anxiety if the increased pain is interpreted as disease progression.

Activity

Watch the following clip 'Hampered by Hormones' from The Prostate Cancer Charity :

http://www.youtube.com/watch?v=5YMhAvwOWr0 (accessed November 2011).

Visit The Prostate Cancer Charity Website and read the *Living with Hormone Therapy* booklet:

http://www.prostate-cancer.org.uk/media/41582/htbooklet.pdf (accessed November 2011).

Make some notes on the main side effects and how you could advise men with prostate cancer to manage these symptoms.

NMC Domain 1: 1.4; 1.5
NMC Domain 2: 2.6
NMC Domain 3: 3.1; 3.2; 3.3; 3.4; 3.5; 3.7; 3.8

Ending treatment

The end of treatment can be a particularly stressful time for a patient and their family. It is a period of uncertainty – Has the treatment worked? What will happen in the future? Will it come back? Who do I talk to if I have a concern?

Many patients feel lost in transition – they are no longer attending hospital regularly and their GP may not know their case very well. The majority will be followed up as an outpatient and their response to treatment will be reviewed. If the treatment was for symptom management, they may be seen more regularly to monitor the effectiveness of treatment and for additional treatment.

A patient may gauge their body's response to treatment subjectively and indicate that their symptoms have improved but this is often difficult to measure. For instance, a patient may feel better and their pain may be reduced, however the cancer may have only shrunk a little or not at all.

The next chapters explore some of the symptoms a patient with cancer may experience, and address the possible outcomes of diagnosis, end of life care and living with and beyond cancer, considering the long-term effects a diagnosis might have on an individual and their family.

References

Goodwin, P.J., Ennis, M., Pritchard, K.I., et al., 1999. Adjuvant treatment and onset of menopause predict weight gain after breast cancer diagnosis. Journal of Clinical Oncology 17, 120–129.

National Institute for Health and Clinical Excellence, 2006. Breast cancer (early) – hormonal treatments: guidance. NICE, London.

Waugh, A., Grant, A., 2010. Ross and Wilson anatomy and physiology in health and illness. Churchill Livingstone, Edinburgh.

Further reading

Ervik, B., Nordoy, T., Asplund, K., 2010. Hit by waves: living with local advanced or localized prostate cancer treated with endocrine therapy or under active surveillance. Cancer Nursing 33 (5), 382–389.

Fenlon, D., 2006. Hormone therapy. In: Kearney, N., Richardson, A. (Eds.), Nursing patients with cancer: principles and practice. Churchill Livingstone, Edinburgh.

Fenlon, D., 2008. Endocrine therapies. In: Corner, J., Bailey, C. (Eds.), Cancer nursing: care in context. 2nd ed. Blackwell, Oxford.

Pennery, E., 2008. The role of endocrine therapies in reducing risk of recurrence in postmenopausal women with hormone receptor-positive breast cancer. European Journal of Oncology Nursing 12 (3), 233–243.

Souhami, R., Tobias, J., 2005. Cancer and its management, 5th ed. Blackwell, Oxford.

Yarbro, C.H., Hansen Frogge, M., Godman, M., 2004. Cancer symptom management. Jones and Bartlett, Boston.

Yarbro, C.H., Hansen Frogge, M., Godman, M., 2005. Cancer nursing: principles and practice, 6th ed. Jones and Bartlett, Boston.

Websites

Breast Cancer Care patient information, http://www.breastcancercare.org.uk/breast-cancer-breast-health/treatment-side-effects/hormone-therapy/ (accessed May 2011).

The Prostate Cancer Charity patient information, http://www.prostate-cancer.org.uk/info/prostate_cancer/treatment_hormones.asp (accessed May 2011).

15

Managing symptoms: assess, plan, implement and evaluate

CHAPTER AIMS

- To introduce the principles of assessment
- To introduce the principles of planning care
- To introduce the principles of managing complex symptoms
- To introduce the principles of evaluating care

Introduction

In any clinical setting you will have the potential to care for a person with a cancer diagnosis who is experiencing one or more of the distressing symptoms explored in this chapter. By engaging in the exercises for each symptom, you are given the opportunity to consider how the symptom can be managed in any specific placement. It is important to apply the principles of assessment and holistic care of a patient introduced below. Patient care must also take into consideration the cultural and ethnic needs of patients and family members. These are explored in more detail in the Chapter 16, however it is important to start to consider the implications as you develop cultural competence in symptom management. This chapter explores some of the principles in supporting a patient with a cancer diagnosis who is experiencing one or more distressing symptom. This can happen during treatment for the cancer, as well as if the patient is in the palliative care stage of the illness. Some symptoms can continue after the patient has completely recovered from the cancer. For example, fatigue or taste changes can sometimes occur following chemotherapy or radiotherapy and may last for many years. Sometimes symptoms can occur as 'acute events' and need to be dealt with swiftly. These include hypercalcaemia and spinal cord compression.

The principles of assessment

From the first time we meet a patient, we can start to gather information to help us in the care we plan and provide. Don't forget we can often have a lot of information about the patient before we even meet them, for example a referral letter from the patient's own doctor, notes from a team discussion, ward handover or the patient's hospital notes. This process of gathering information about a patient is called 'assessment'. Data can be gathered from a variety of sources and this is the basis for our actions and decisions. It is important to remember that assessment is an ongoing process rather than one point of interaction.

The nursing process (Roper et al 2000) suggests assessment is the 'first step' in the four-step cycle of planning, implementing and evaluating care. Uys and Habermann (2005) recognise the importance of collecting information in the assessment process, while Holland et al (2008) refer to assessment as a 'cyclical activity' that includes collecting and reviewing information and linking this assessment to impact on activities of living.

The assessment process is just part of the care planning pathway and it is essential that all information gathered is correct and communicated to the appropriate team members at the appropriate time.

Remember, the information we gather includes that from the patient, family *and* professional teams.

 Activity

List the ways we can gather information about a patient, considering the following themes:

- What we see.
- What we smell.
- What we hear.
- What we read.
- What we are told.

How much of this list is information that is routinely included in patient admission documentation? Look at the things in your list that are not routinely documented. Prepare to discuss with your mentor how this information might be recorded.

NMC Domain 1: 1.1; 1.3
NMC Domain 3: 3.1; 3.3

The principles of planning care

When we have gathered information about a patient, we are then able to plan the care we are going to provide. It is important that any information is clarified and communicated with wider team members in an appropriate way. Remember that any information we have about a patient is confidential and must be respected and kept safe at all times. The NMC code of conduct (NMC 2008) states confidentiality as a patient's right so, as you gather information, it is important to inform patients how this will be used. Doing this shows the patient respect.

One way to collate this information in a logical and holistic way is by using the Roper, Logan and Tierney model (Roper et al 2000) (Figs 15.1 and 15.2). This model was originally developed in 1980 by Nancy Roper and published under the title *The Elements of Nursing* and is a collection of core themes around activities of living. They were developed with the idea that activities of living can be applied to patients in any clinical area, are patient focused and can give a clear idea of the needs of a patient and their family at any point in time. You may have already seen this model used in a previous practice placement. Sometimes they are referred to as the activities of daily living (ADLs). Admission assessment forms for both acute hospitals and community settings are often based on this model.

There are 12 activities of living which take a holistic approach:

1. Maintaining a safe environment.
2. Communicating.
3. Breathing.
4. Eating and drinking.
5. Eliminating.
6. Personal cleansing and dressing.
7. Controlling body temperature.
8. Mobilising.

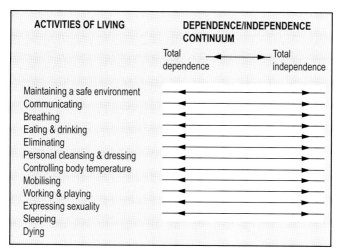

Fig 15.1 The Roper, Logan and Tierney model (Roper et al 2000)

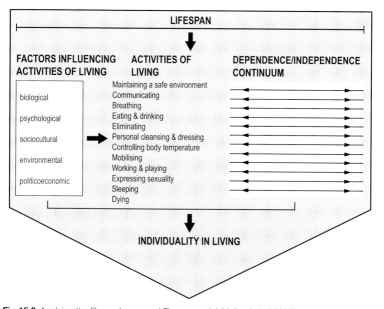

Fig 15.2 Applying the Roper, Logan and Tierney model (Holland et al 2008)

9. Working and playing.
10. Expressing sexuality.
11. Sleeping.
12. Dying.

 Activity

> Find out about the admission model used in your practice placement. Look out for the activities of living. These are sometimes called the activities of daily living. Familiarise yourself with this model so when you meet your first patient on placement, you can already be gathering important information needed to plan and provide their care.
>
> NMC Domain 1: 1.1; 1.2; 1.5
> NMC Domain 2: 2.7
> NMC Domain 3: 3.1; 3.3

These activities of living are not separate themes but are linked through biological, psychosocial and political factors. Each of the activities are interlinked and will impact on a person's degree of dependence or independence (Holland et al 2008).

 Activity

> Spend some time considering these 12 activities of living from the Roper, Logan and Tierney model. Consider how you achieve your own activities of daily living. How important are each one to you? What things can impact on how you achieve these activities of living? For example, normal patterns of eating and drinking may be affected if you are working night shifts. Consider what impact this may have on your life and wellbeing.
>
> NMC Domain 1: 1.2; 1.3
> NMC Domain 3.1; 3.3

Collecting information from a family member is called a family assessment. Some specialist units will have a specific assessment form for a family assessment which can include questions about knowledge of a patient's diagnosis, feelings about this diagnosis, how the family is coping and any dependants, for example children, adolescents, pets or other ill family members.

Gathering information about a patient and their family is not easy. There are many things that can hinder the effective collection of data and this can have a direct impact on the care given or understanding of what the priority needs are for a patient and their family. Information can be gathered about a patient at admission (part 1). If the patient dies, part 2 can be completed about what happened at the time of death and how the family reacted. This information can help with planning ongoing bereavement support (See Appendix 2).

Remember, information gathered is only as good as the process of documenting and communicating this information to the appropriate person at the appropriate time.

Problems are often encountered in gathering assessment information. Knowing something about a patient and not passing it on may have a big impact on how their individual care needs are met. For example, a patient might tell you that his sense of taste has changed since chemotherapy, but he doesn't like to tell his wife since she will get upset if he can't taste the food she cooks him. Consider why this information might be important. If the patient becomes more poorly, feels nauseated and goes off his food, tempting him to eat is going to be a really important care intervention by both the professional team and his wife. If he can't taste, this may be more challenging to achieve. Addressing such issues is harder for a patient, family and care team when the patient is not feeling well or if the patient is deteriorating.

Activity

Read through the following scenario and consider the information you have about the patient:

■ You are helping to care for a man who has been admitted from another ward in the hospital and you have been invited to go with the staff nurse on the ward round.

■ In this morning's evaluation of patient care, the following has been written by the night staff:

06.35. Poor night's sleep, awake since 3 am. Seemed to settle after a cup of tea. No complaints of pain.

■ The doctor says to the patient, '*I hear you are not sleeping*'. The patient answers '*No Doctor*'.

■ On the ward round, the doctors discuss a prescription for sleeping tablets.

■ On the activities of living admission sheet, the following is written:

Sleeping: no problems, sleep pattern not changed for years

■ You were on a late shift last night and overheard a conversation between this patient and the waitress who was serving the evening drinks:

My sleep isn't good. I normally go to bed sometime after midnight and sleep for about 3 hours, then lots of waking and dosing. Been like this for years since I was a night shift worker. Is it all right on this ward to put my little light on and ask for a cup of tea in the night?

Consider the information we have about this patient, his sleep pattern and his current needs.

Here is a list of what we already know about the patient:

1. He has a long-term sleep pattern that has not changed for several years.

2. He is open with this information with some members of the care team.

3. He appears reluctant to freely offer information to the doctor.

4. Having a cup of tea in the night seems to help him feel settled.

Where can other information be found?

1. Admission notes from his previous ward and possible previous admissions.

2. A conversation with the patient to ask what his sleep pattern means to him. Is it a problem? What helps?

Consider what information is important and what the doctor needs to know to ensure safe and appropriate treatment is prescribed.

Questions to consider:

1. Is he waking because it is his normal routine?

2. Is he waking because he is in a new environment?

3. Is he waking because he is in pain or experiencing another form of distress?

It is important to remember not to make the assumption that he is waking out of habit. Ongoing assessment of the patient ensures symptoms are not overlooked and his needs are appropriately met.

NMC Domain 1: 1.1; 1.3
NMC Domain 2: 2.1; 2.2; 2.3
NMC Domain 3: 3.1; 3.3; 3.4

Remember, admission sheets can have information added during the patient stay by any member of the care team. Building up information about a patient and their family is a form of ongoing assessment.

The principles of managing common symptoms experienced by cancer and palliative care patients

Understanding the causes of symptoms and treatment options available is an important part of the assessment and care planning process. We now introduce you to some common symptoms experienced by cancer and palliative care patients and offer explanations about possible causes as well as some care interventions.

When managing complex symptoms, it is important to remember the core principles of assessment, planning and evaluation. This can be done simply by using the 'three Cs' model:

- *Communication*: this includes the information gathering phase and involves how information about the patient is communicated with the patient as well as other members of the care team. Understanding what the key issues are, discussing treatment options and communicating options is the first stage in ensuring care planned considers *all* the important factors that are relevant to the patient.
- *Choice*: giving information to the patient about what is happening is essential for the patient to make an informed choice about treatment. This includes the concept of consent and is one of the underpinning ethical principles of autonomy. To refresh your knowledge of ethical principles, go back to Chapter 5.

If patients feel they have choices in their treatment regimen, they are more likely be compliant with taking medication, attending appointments, etc. For example, if a patient understands the link between a specific medication and risk of constipation, they are more likely to take the prescribed laxatives.

- *Care*: this must be planned, holistic and patient centred. Attention to detail is vital. Care must be continually evaluated by all members of the multidisciplinary team, documented and then renegotiated with the patient and family. Always consider the needs of patients.

 Activity

Under each of the 'three C' headings, list all the activities you can undertake as a nurse to ensure principles of symptom management are achieved. To help you do this, reflect back on the observations you have made in current and previous placements. To refresh your knowledge of the principles of assessment, go back to page 129.

Good symptom management relies on an effective assessment process.

NMC Domain 1: 1.1; 1.5; 1.7

Pain: causes, assessment and management

A universally accepted definition of pain is that it is an unpleasant sensory and emotional experience that is associated with actual or potential tissue damage (International Association for the Study of Pain 2007). Pain is complex and understanding what is both initiating the pain and maintaining it is important for effective management. Chapter 5 on palliative care introduced you to the concept of 'total pain'. The contemporary way of referring to total pain is from a 'biopsychosocial' perspective (Holdcroft & Power 2003) and can be divided into three factors:

1. The person – includes biological and psychological influences.
2. Type of disease – includes past history and present disease.
3. Environment – includes cultural expectations, upbringing, roles, lifestyle.

The most challenging part of managing pain is the subjectivity of pain; what it means to one person is different from another person, as is the individual's ability to manage the pain. 'Pain is whatever the person experiencing it says it is, existing whenever he says it does' (McCaffery 1968:95). While this work of McCaffery is old, it continues to be a fundamental principle of pain management.

A simple way of developing our understanding of normal pain transmission is to consider it from the following four perspectives:

1. Transduction – involves the process of converting mechanical, thermal or chemical noxious or painful stimulus into a nervous impulse.
2. Transmission – involves the nervous impulse being conducted by sensory nerves to the central nervous system. Different nerves carry different impulses.
3. Perception – conscious perception of pain is perceived by an individual once all the incoming nervous messages are interpreted by the brain.
4. Modulation – throughout the process, various physiological and psychological mechanisms can adjust the nociceptive message to either increase or decrease the pain experienced.

Activity

Re-read the notes you made about your personal experiences of pain on page 39. Now consider how you might know a patient is in pain. Make a list of

the words that a person might use to describe pain followed by a list of the behaviours you might observe. Consider how this information might have been gathered and be documented in the patient's case notes and communicated across the care team.

NMC Domain 1: 1.1
NMC Domain 2: 2.4
NMC Domain 3: 3.2; 3.7

Types of pain

Table 15.1 gives a simple overview of two types of pain, the basic physiology and words associated with how pain might be experienced.

Activity

Using Table 15.1, write a few sentences about the impact the different types of pain can have on the activities of living.

To help you do this, you might want to refer back to pain lecture notes from your course. If this is a new subject to you, look at the recommended physiology text for your course and read about pain and pain pathways. Make notes on the new words or phrases you come across to help to retain knowledge and understanding.

NMC Domain 1: 1.1; 1.2;
NMC Domain 2: 2.2; 2.4
NMC Domain 3: 3.2

Doing the above exercise helps link the physiology of the origins of pain and the impact pain can have on holistic wellbeing. This way of thinking starts the assessment process and is the first step

Table 15.1 Types of pain

Type of pain	Physiology	Description	Examples
Nociceptive pain: Visceral (pain in an internal organ) Somatic (pain of the musculoskeletal system)	Pain is caused when sensory receptors (nerve endings) become activated by damage or injury sending pain messages to the central nervous system Can be referred pain Usually well localised and the patient can point with one finger to the location of their pain	Cramping Squeezing Pressure Sharp Intermittent Aching Deep Dull Gnawing Throbbing	Myocardial infarction (heart attack) Kidney stone Bowel obstruction, gall stones Pressure from within or on a visceral organ Cut Peritonitis Bone metastases Sprained ankle Toothache Burn Outside force, e.g. a punch
Neuropathic pain	Pain that arises from damage to sensory nerves by disease or a specific event which changes the messages sent to the central nervous system Neuropathic pain is defined by the International Association for the Study of Pain as pain arising as a direct consequence of a lesion or disease affecting the somatosensory system	Burning Electric shocks Pins and needles Stabbing Shooting Feels like an 'electric shock'	Associated with wide variety of chronic diseases: diabetes, carpal nerve entrapment, sciatica, spinal cord injury, neuralgia

in the effective management of pain and is where the understanding of biopsychsocial factors for a holistic approach is important.

Assessing pain correctly is fundamental to ensuring analgesia prescribed is appropriate and effective. Asking how the pain is and getting the patient to describe the pain is a useful way to establish possible causes. Also finding out what makes it worse and what makes it better is important too. The assessment tool in Figure 15.3 is called the Brief Pain Inventory (BPI) and is used in many clinical areas and is a quick way to explore pain with a patient.

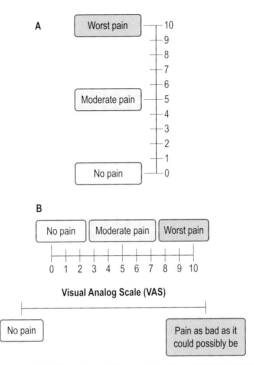

Fig 15.3 Pain assessment tool (reproduced with permission from McCaffery M, Pasero C (1999) Pain, clinical manual, 2nd edn. Mosby, St Louis)

Activity

Find out how the nurses in your practice placement assess a patient's pain. If a pain assessment tool is used, how often is it completed? How is the information communicated with the healthcare team? How often is a patient's pain reviewed?

NMC Domain 1: 1.5
NMC Domain 2.2; 2.7
NMC Domain 3.1; 3.3

Management of pain

Once pain is effectively assessed, appropriate analgesia can be prescribed. Often a patient may have analgesia prescribed 'as required' or 'prn'. The potential problem with this is it is reliant on the care team noticing the person is in pain or the patient asking for analgesia. Literature suggests this is something that healthcare professionals do not always do well and patients may not always feel able to ask. It is also important to record if any 'as required' analgesia given has helped to relieve the pain. This can be done by returning to the

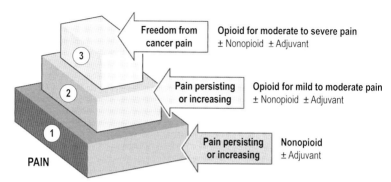

Fig 15.4 WHO analgesic step ladder (WHO (1996) Cancer pain relief, 2nd edn. WHO, Geneva)

patient within half an hour of giving the analgesia. If analgesia is not relieving pain, it needs to be reviewed by the care team. If several 'as required' drugs are given over a period of time with good effect, these should be converted into regular administration. The plan of care should aim for the patient being pain free and not routinely needing 'as required' medications.

The World Health Organisation (WHO) analgesic step ladder is shown in Figure 15.4. Here we can see that analgesia is staged from a non-opioid, to a weak opioid and then to a strong opioid. This is the recommended ladder by which analgesia is prescribed.

Sometimes morphine analgesia is not prescribed or given 'as required' (prn) for fear it will harm the patient. Equally, this may be the reason a patient may refuse to take analgesia or admit to being in pain. An article which will help you to understand this issue in more depth is Stannard (2008) (see References).

Non-drug interventions for pain can be really helpful to patients. These can be done even before a registered nurse is needed to get a prescription. If a patient is in pain, ask where the pain is and what normally helps that pain. They might say 'sitting up' or 'massaging my legs' or 'a cup of tea'. These interventions can help bring down a patient's pain score. Always remember to document any non-drug interventions you do.

Remember, effective management of pain relies on comprehensive assessment of the whole person throughout the time you care for them.

Activity

When you are in your practice placement area, have a look at two or three patient drug cards. Find out if each patient is prescribed any analgesia and, if so, see how their prescription relates to the WHO analgesic step ladder. If the step ladder was not followed, consider why this might be. Do you have enough history about the patient to be able to answer this question? Consider what additional information would be helpful for you. Remember that gathering information about a patient is vital for managing symptoms effectively.

NMC Domain 1: 1.1; 1.2
NMC Domain 2: 2.7
NMC Domain 3: 3.1; 3.2; 3.3
NMC Domain 4: 4.2

Nausea and vomiting

The symptoms of nausea and vomiting are often associated together, bit this is not the right approach. It is important to consider the causes and management of nausea as separate to the causes and management of vomiting. Some patients will have both symptoms. Forty-two percent of patients with cancer have just nausea at some point while 32% have both nausea and vomiting together (Twycross et al 2009).

Nausea and vomiting can be caused by a wide range of factors, so understanding physiological processes is an important part of being able to gather the correct information in the assessment process. In the brain, there are specific areas that provoke the vomiting response: the vomiting centre and chemoreceptor trigger zone (CTZ) in the medulla oblongata, which is at the base of the brain, the cerebral cortex and the vestibular centre. In addition, right through the gastrointestinal tract there are peripheral pathways where receptors send messages via the vagus nerve to the brain to activate the CTZ and vomiting centre. Figure 15.5 is a simple diagram demonstrating how the pathways work.

There are seven core causes of vomiting, often referred to as vomiting pathways or syndromes. We now look at each in turn to explain what causes the vomiting and to understand treatment options:

1. Raised intracranial pressure: if intracranial pressure is raised, this will stimulate the vomiting centre which produces histamines. Effective management is to use antihistamines to reduce the histamines collecting in the vomiting centre.
2. Irritation of the visceral and gastrointestinal serosa, the lining of the gastrointestinal wall which secretes fluid to keep the bowel wall lubricated: once irritated, the peripheral nerves activate the vagus nerve to stimulate the vomiting centre.
3. Gastric stasis/gastric outlet obstruction: if the contents of the stomach or intestine become static or are obstructed, the peripheral nerves are stimulated to send messages via the vagus nerve to the vomiting centre. Stasis and obstruction can be caused by cancer or medication that slows down bowel movements, for example diamorphine.
4. Oesophageal obstruction: this can be caused directly by cancer, oral thrush or painful swallowing (odynophagia). As well as a stimulation of the vomiting centre by the peripheral nerves in the gastrointestinal tract, the flow of saliva can be increased. If this becomes a problem for the patient, medication can be prescribed to reduce saliva flow.
5. Pharyngeal stimulation: this can be caused by excessive sputum or oral thrush. Reducing histamines in the vomiting centre can relieve nausea.
6. Chemically-induced nausea: this can range from poisons to chemotherapy which stimulate the CTZ. Once stimulated, it will stimulate the vomiting centre.
7. Anxiety/anticipatory nausea/vomiting: this cause of vomiting is sometimes associated with anticipatory vomiting in patients who are waiting for a cycle of chemotherapy. Anxiety about the disease process, treatments, hospital admissions and psychosocial factors can all lead to nausea or/and vomiting. Giving the patient reassurance and medication to reduce anxiety can help to relieve nausea/vomiting.

Understanding the physiology of vomiting pathways is the first step in assessment of nausea and/or vomiting. The specific treatment and care will depend on the cause(s). Table 15.2 links the vomiting pathways/syndromes to potential treatment options and nursing care and interventions.

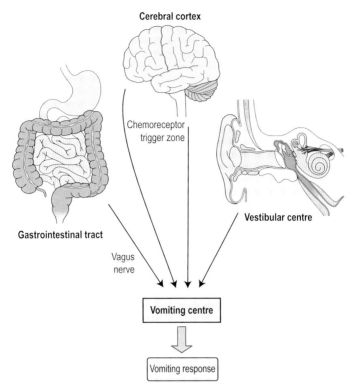

Cerebral cortex

Chemoreceptor
trigger zone

Vestibular centre

Gastrointestinal tract

Vagus
nerve

Vomiting centre

Vomiting response

Fig 15.5 Vomiting pathways (adapted from: Campbell T, Hately J (2000) The management of nausea and vomiting in advanced cancer. International Journal of Palliative Nursing 6(1):18–25)

Activity

List all the team members who you think might be involved in supporting a patient with nausea, vomiting or both. Find out how many of these team members are available in your practice placement. Find out from your mentor how a referral is made to a team member who is *not* working daily in the practice placement environment.

Using the *British National Formulary* (BNF), find out a bit more about antiemetic drugs used for the different pathways. Look under 'antiemetic', 'dopamine antagonist' and 'antihistamine and anxiolytic'. Jot down notes for each drug and link to the appropriate pathways using Table 15.2.

Remember that a patient who is vomiting can be given subcutaneous injections. Ideally these should be continued for 3 days of non-vomiting, then given orally (Twycross et al 2009).

NMC Domain 1: 1.5; 1.6
NMC Domain 2: 2.1; 2.2; 2.7
NMC Domain 3: 3.2
NMC Domain 4: 4.6

Table 15.2 Vomiting syndromes and the management of nausea

Syndrome	Vomiting Pathway	Clinical Features	Causes	Antiemetic	Adjuvent interventions and nursing care
1. Raised Intracranial pressure/ meningism	Vomiting centre via cerebral cortex	Neurological signs e.g. papilloedema, drowsiness, dizziness, headache, nausea /vomiting	Cerebral tumour Intracranial tumour Intracranial bleeding Infiltration of the meninges by tumour Skull metastases Cerebral infection	Antihistamine e.g. cyclizine	High dose steroids may reduce cerebral oedema and/or tumour mass
2. Irritation of the visceral and gastrointestinal serosa	Vomiting centre Gastrointestinal tract via vegus nerve	Pain Colic Altered bowel habit Nausea Vomiting of faecal fluid in obstruction	Liver metastases Ureteric obstruction Tumour Constipation Bowel obstruction Lymph nodes	Antihistamine e.g. cyclizine	Relieve the cause e.g. treat the constipation with stimulant laxatives and enemas as required Consider steroid therapy for reduction of peri-tumour oedema

Continued

Table 15.2 Vomiting syndromes and the management of nausea—cont'd

Syndrome	Vomiting Pathway	Clinical Features	Causes	Antiemetic	Adjuvent interventions and nursing care
3. Gastric stasis/ gastric outflow obstruction	Vomiting centre Gastrointestinal tract	Epigrastric fullness/ discomfort Flatulence Hiccough Acid reflux Gastric regurgitation Nausea often relieved by vomiting	Anti-cholinergic drugs Autonomic failure Ascites Hepatomegaly Tumour infiltration Peptic ulcer Gastritis	Prokinetic e.g. metoclopramide	Review drug regime Dietary advice – small amounts often Paracentisis for ascites
4. Oesophageal obstruction	Vomiting centre	Retching Nausea	Tumour growth Oesophageal thrush Odynophagia (painful swelling) Chemotherapy antibiotics	Antihistamine e.g. cyclizine	Oral hygiene Treat oral candidosis e.g. nystatin
5. Pharyngeal stimulation	Vomiting centre	Retching Nausea	Excessive sputum Oral thrush	Antihistamine e.g. cyclizine	Oral hygiene Treat oral candidosis e.g. nystatin

Table 15.2 Vomiting syndromes and the management of nausea—cont'd

Syndrome	Vomiting Pathway	Clinical Features	Causes	Antiemetic	Adjuvent interventions and nursing care
6. Chemically induced nausea	Chemoreceptor Trigger Zone (CTZ)	Nausea and retching more than vomiting. Vomiting does not relieve the vomiting. Nausea is usually constant Features a specific drug toxicity.	Drugs. e.g. chemotherapy opiates, anticonvulsants digoxin Metabolic e.g hypercalcaemia, uraemia, liver failure Toxins e.g.	Dopamine antagonist e.g. haloperidol, domperidone, metoclopramide 5HT3 antagonist ondansetron, granisetron NK1 receptor antagonist e.g aprepitant	Review drug management Check biochemistry Treat underlying cause e.g. hypercalcaemia
7. Anxiety	Vomiting centre via cerebral cortex	Nausea Waves of nausea and vomiting Distraction may relieve symptoms	Psychological and emotional distress Anticipating emesis with chemotherapy	Antihistamine Anticholinergics	Address anxiety with reassurance and psychological techniques Relaxation Benzodiazepines e.g lorazepam Ensure adequate pain control

Adapted from Campbell T, Hately J (2000) The management of nausea and vomiting in advanced cancer. International Journal of Palliative Nursing 6(1) 18-25

*Non-medication care of the patient
who is experiencing nausea
or/and vomiting*

Supporting a patient who has nausea or/and vomiting must not just be through giving medication. Ensuring privacy, mouth washes and vomit bowls is essential. Also consider if the environment is calm and free of strong smells. Remember that nauseated patients can be particularly sensitive to perfumes and fragranced body wash. Check what they want to use and be careful what you wear yourself. Cooled fizzy drinks can be offered and make sure these are renewed regularly. Relatives can also be supported to understand what to do and not do to help relieve nausea and vomiting.

Consider anticipatory vomiting. Sight and smell of food can often exacerbate the distress. Ask the patient if this is a problem – they might like their curtains closed during meal times. Well-meaning relatives may be talking about food to tempt them, making the feelings worse, or bringing food to the bedside.

Ensure the ward waitress knows what to offer the patient. Serving portions on a side plate can make a meal suddenly appear appetising rather than daunting.

Constipation

Half of the people diagnosed with cancer experience a change in their bowel habits leading to constipation (Twycross et al 2009). One in six of these will class this as severe and it is the most common reported gastrointestinal problem. Constipation is defined as the passage of hard, dry stools with excessive straining and decrease in frequency (Doyle et al 2005). How we define normal bowel movement is determined by the patient and their normal pattern. Taking a comprehensive history of bowel movements, and when changes have occurred in the past, can help with management.

Constipation is common in patients receiving analgesic medication. It is essential that anyone prescribed an opioid also have a laxative prescribed. This is because opioids have a direct effect on the smooth muscle of the large intestine and slow down peristaltic movement. This means that more water is absorbed from the large intestine.

Activity

Make notes about the potential causes of constipation under the following headings:
- Lifestyle.
- Medication.
- Disease process.
- Previous history.

NMC Domain 1: 1.2
NMC Domain 2: 2.6
NMC Domain 3: 3.1; 3.2

Oral care

Maintaining a healthy mouth is a fundamental part of nursing care and essentially an important focus of care for cancer patients. A mouth is kept clean and healthy by having a good diet, adequate flow of saliva, mastication (chewing food) and oral cleaning.

A good diet can be hindered by a patient having surgery, being nauseated, loss of appetite, dysphagia (difficulty swallowing) or being in the last days of life.

Mastication can be altered by having ill-fitting dentures/no dentures, surgery or lethargy. A patient can be encouraged to take a healthy diet by chopping food, or a soft diet if mastication is a problem. This is particularly helpful as well if the patient is suffering with fatigue.

Activity

Consider how you naturally maintain a healthy mouth. List your thoughts under each of the following headings:

- Good diet.
- Adequate saliva flow.
- Mastication.
- Oral cleaning.

You might need to refresh your knowledge of mouth anatomy and physiology from your lecture notes to complete this exercise. If you have not had a lecture yet, consult a core anatomy and physiology textbook, either one that has been recommended by your training school or, alternatively, a textbook such as Clancy and McVicar (2009) (see References).

NMC Domain 1: 1.3; 1.4
NMC Domain 2: 2.6
NMC Domain 3: 3.2

A reduced flow of saliva is experienced by up to 90% of patients with cancer. This can happen during and following radiotherapy and chemotherapy and the use of many medications, for example morphine. Facial oxygen therapy can also drastically reduce saliva. Saliva is important since it breaks down bacteria in the mouth and protects the mouth from extreme temperatures. Artificial saliva is often prescribed and oxygen can be given nasally or humidified.

Oral cleaning can be affected if a patient has bleeding or sore gums. This is seen frequently in patients receiving chemotherapy or with a low platelet count. Patients with an impaired gag reflex may feel frightened of choking.

A clean healthy mouth is essential in reducing the risk of a patient developing thrush. This is an oral fungal infection called *Candida albicans* which is present in the mouth of about 50% of people. It becomes a problem if the chemistry of the oral cavity changes. Early assessment by taking a history and detecting new problems are important to establish how care can be prioritised and planned (Piper 2008). Many patients may have had poor mouth hygiene prior to their illness; for others, problems are new and distressing. Sorting out poor-fitting dentures early on can prevent a severely sore mouth developing as the disease progresses.

 Activity

Look up the following terms associated with oral hygiene and write down nursing interventions to support a patient:

- Stomatitis.
- Gingivitis.
- Xerostomia.
- Oral *Candia albicans*.

NMC Domain 3: 3.1; 3.2; 3.3; 3.7

Fatigue

Cancer-related fatigue is the most common symptom experienced by patients receiving cancer treatments (Ahlberg et al 2003) and is described as 'a persistent, subjective sense of tiredness related to cancer or cancer treatment that interferes with usual functioning' (Mock et al 2005:1). The incidence of cancer-related fatigue is high – 82% of people with a cancer diagnosis will experience fatigue for a few days per month (Stone et al 2000). So it is very likely you will nurse a person with fatigue in this practice placement.

When a patient experiences fatigue, they may not say 'I am feeling fatigued today'. Instead, they may use a variety of other words: I am tired; I can't be bothered; I don't want visitors; I can't stand the noise; I don't want to eat; I can't brush my hair; I am too tired to sleep. Patients may also indicate fatigue not just by what they say, but how they look and behave. For example, you might notice a woman who, on admission, wore make up but is now not interested in her lipstick or renewing her nail varnish. Or a family member might tell you they are worried about their dad because he is not shaving.

Another definition of fatigue suggests it is a 'subjective unpleasant symptom which incorporates total body feelings ranging from tiredness to exhaustion, creating an unrelenting overall condition which interferes with the individuals' ability to function to their normal capacity' (Ream & Richardson 1996:527). This definition gives a clearer idea of the impact fatigue may have on activities of living and a person's capacity to maintain normality. It is one of the first definitions of fatigue and continues to be one of the core understandings on which contemporary care is planned and delivered.

Not understanding fatigue can potentially lead to emotional and psychosocial distress that can exacerbate other symptoms, making all of them more difficult to manage effectively. Understanding fatigue can be a particular challenge for family members. Part of the definition of palliative care is to keep the dying process normal. By recognising the impact of fatigue, it is possible to work with the patient and their family to keep as much normality as possible.

There are many causes of fatigue and a patient can have just one or many interacting together. This is why fatigue can be such a complex problem to effectively manage. Fatigue during and following both chemotherapy and radiotherapy is very common. It can also occur due to the cancer growing, infections, pain, medication, co-morbidities and anxiety/depression.

Often fatigue and depression are interlinked (O'Regan & Hegarty 2009) and management needs to focus on both aspects of care.

Factors that can contribute to fatigue include inactivity, deconditioning, poor diet, poor sleep, changes in routine and anxiety about the disease process.

🔖 Activity

Using the Roper, Logan and Tierney model, consider how fatigue may impact on each activity of living. Go through each of the activities and consider what might make the fatigue worse and what might help the fatigue.

Now consider the impact of fatigue on the wellbeing of patients and the challenges this presents to the care team.

To develop an understanding of the impact of fatigue on the holistic wellbeing of patients, read the article by O'Regan and Hegarty (2009) (see References).

NMC Domain 1: 1.2
NMC Domain 2: 2.7
NMC Domain 3: 3.1; 3.2; 3.7; 3.9

Body image and altered body image

How we view our own body is important since it is the way we tell ourselves how we look to others. This image of self is the mental picture we have of ourself but is not necessarily the way other people see us. A change in the mental picture of self can have a big impact on how we view what is happening. For example, a woman receiving chemotherapy may lose her hair and this can impact on how she views herself. It is important to be aware that anticipation of a change in body image can start at diagnosis, well before treatment begins (Frith et al 2007). A change in one's perception of body image is called 'altered body image' and is a complex symptom to manage. Altered body image can be temporary or permanent, depending on the causes and the person's ability to cope with the change (Salter 1997). Often, altered body image becomes a problem because the patient does not have the ability to cope with the changes or because of the behaviour of others towards them (Price 2000). This can include lack of support, help and information from healthcare professionals who often fail to acknowledge the importance of how patients view themselves.

When supporting a patient with altered body image, it is important to show you are interested on how *they* view their body. If a person is distressed at their loss of weight, it is not helpful to dismiss this concern by saying 'you look just fine'. Instead we need to find out what this loss of weight might mean to *them*. It might mean they can no longer wear favourite clothes, they may feel a loss of their sexuality or concern that it is a sign the cancer is progressing.

 Activity

Consider the impact society can have on body image. Start by considering what impacts on how you view yourself.

Now look through some magazines. Count how many times image is raised: in adverts, articles, pictures, comments. How important is image in these magazines? What is seen to be normal? Consider how a person who has had disfiguring surgery, loss of hair, gained weight or lost part of their body function may feel looking at these magazines.

NMC Domain 1: 1.2; 1.3; 1.4
NMC Domain 2: 2.3; 2.6
NMC Domain 4.4

Once we start to understand what altered body image means to a patient, we are in a position to offer support strategies and plan focused and appropriate care.

To explore further the impact of weight loss associated with advancing cancer on body image, read the article by Hinsley and Hughes (2007) (see References).

Breathlessness

Breathlessness is the 'subjective experience of breathing discomfort' (Twycross et al 2009:145). The distress a patient feels is individual to that person and does not always correspond to how we might view their breathlessness. A lot of anxiety and fear is associated with both the onset of breathlessness or worry that it will get worse. Breathlessness can be caused by a primary lung cancer, lung metastasis, respiratory muscle weakness or fluid within the lung cavity. This is called a pleural effusion and you may see a patient regularly returning to hospital to have the fluid removed from the lung; a pleural aspiration. Recurring effusions can be a sign of advancing disease. Pain, fatigue and anxiety can exacerbate the feelings of breathlessness and have a great impact on a person's ability to undertake their activities of living.

The clinical management of breathlessness is divided into two specific areas – for patients breathless at rest and for patients breathless on exertion. It is important to be clear about which type of breathlessness the patient has before an effective treatment regimen can be planned. The assessment process will help with this.

 Activity

Revisit the activities of living outlined on pages 130–132. Consider the impact breathlessness may have on each of these activities. Make a list of the care interventions that can help relieve breathlessness and limit distress for:

– a patient at rest

– a patient on exertion.

Don't forget to consider the impact on the family too.

Remember that the Roper, Logan and Tierney model is an effective assessment tool for a specific symptom on which to be able to plan care.

NMC Domain 1: 1.1; 1.2
NMC Domain 2: 2.4
NMC Domain 3: 3.1; 3.2

Psychological distress

In Chapter 5, we introduced the concept of psychological distress when exploring the definition of palliative care. Also, we have considered the wellbeing of patients when looking at the activities of living. It is important to remember that a patient can experience a wide range of distressing feelings and emotions at any stage of the cancer journey. Providing support at all stages of this journey is an important part of nursing care. Awareness of the potential for distress and being able to recognise the signs is an important part of providing holistic care. Distress is often linked to the term 'suffering' and you will often hear the two linked. The degree of suffering or distress is not directly linked to the diagnosis or specific symptoms but more to how a particular patient associates meaning to what is happening (Payne et al 2008).

As nurses, we cannot always prevent suffering or psychological distress. Recognising the links between the two is the first step in being able to effectively support both the patient and their relatives. It is important to allow patients to express their feelings of distress, so they can be supported to work through their feelings of suffering. They may then be able to develop strength or resilience to help them face what the cancer diagnosis and treatment options may bring. Involving family and friends is really important. Often they feel helpless and distressed themselves when they see a person they care for so ill and unhappy. Encouraging patients and relatives to express these feelings helps to develop the therapeutic relationships (Burzotta & Noble 2010) essential in providing holistic care.

The principles of good psychological care include listening to patients and giving priority to what is distressing them most. By showing an interest in their story, we can create a safe place for them to express thoughts and feelings. This may help to give patients some control back to make decisions, helping to reduce feelings of loss. This is also an important part of developing a therapeutic relationship. Being aware of the potential barriers to providing psychological care for a person who is distressed is important. Read the Burzotta and Noble (2010) article which explores barriers in more detail. Make some notes about how these barriers might be reduced from the perspective of your current clinical placement.

Activity

Think about how you might respond to a person who is showing signs of suffering or psychological distress. To help you with this activity you may wish to refer back to the distress thermometer assessment tool introduced on page 35. First, list the ways in which you might know they are distressed. Now make a list of how you might be able to respond to that distress. To help you with this list, use the following headings:

■ Verbal.
■ Non-verbal.
■ Team approach.

NMC Domain 1: 1.5; 1.6
NMC Domain 2: 2.3; 2.4
NMC Domain 3: 3.3

We now look at two symptoms that are often referred to as acute events. They need to be managed quickly to ensure minimal distress for the patient and their family.

Spinal cord compression

Abnormal pressure on the spinal cord is commonly referred to as spinal cord compression (SCC) and is seen predominantly in patients with advanced cancer. Compression can be caused directly or indirectly due to the spread of the cancer, often referred to as metastatic spinal cord compression (MSCC). Metastasis of the spinal column occurs in 3–5% of all patients with cancer (National Collaborating Centre for Cancer 2008). Figure 15.6 illustrates the MSCC of compression along the spinal cord.

Growth of the cancer can cause pressure or bleeding, affecting nerves around the spinal cord. It can also be caused or made worse by localised infection. Patients with MSCC may be receiving active chemotherapy or radiotherapy treatments. Alternatively, they may be in the palliative stage of their illness. For a more detailed explanation of the impact of a spinal cord compression, read the article by Drudge-Coates and Rajbabul (2008a).

Rapid assessment, diagnosis and management are vital for *both* groups

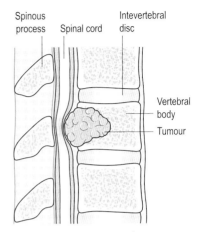

Fig 15.6 Spinal cord compression

of patients since the priority of care is to manage pain and prevent irreversible paralysis. Once paralysis has occurred, it usually cannot be reversed. Research shows that if a patient has the ability to walk at the time of diagnosis of MSCC, they are more likely to walk following treatment (Drudge-Coates & Rajbabul 2008b). Also, being mobile at the time of diagnosis indicates a better overall outcome following treatment (Levack et al 2001). Often immobility can start due to the onset of pain weeks or months before weakness occurs. MSCC is most common in patients diagnosed with breast, lung, prostate and thyroid cancer; in these patients, the incidence may be as high as 19% (National Collaborating Centre for Cancer 2008).

Table 15.3 compares prognosis for a number of spinal cord compression factors.

The position of compression on the spine determines the symptoms patients experience (Fig. 15.7).

Table 15.3 Spinal cord compression factors (National Collaborating Centre for Cancer 2008:40)

Good prognosis	Poor prognosis
Breast cancer as the primary site	Lung or melanoma primary
Solitary or few spinal metastases	Multiple spinal metastases
Absence of visceral metastases	Visceral metastases
Ability to walk aided or unaided	Unable to walk
Minimal neurological impairment	Severe weakness
No previous radiotherapy	Recurrence after radiotherapy

Accurate assessment is important in diagnosing MSCC. Low back pain is commonly the first symptom, occurring in 95% of patients, with weakness of limbs occurring in 85% of patients (Levack et al 2001). Changes in sensation are common and include numbness of the fingers and toes. It is also important to remember that a diagnosis if MSCC can be the first time a patient is aware that he/she has a diagnosis of cancer – 23% of patients diagnosed with MSCC have no prior cancer diagnosis (National Collaborating Centre for Cancer 2008).

Rapid management of a patient with MSCC is a priority. Once diagnosis is made, steroids may be started to reduce localised inflammation, and radiotherapy over 2 to 4 weeks often works well to alleviate pain. If a patient is well enough, surgery to relieve the pressure and stabilise the spine is the treatment of choice, however often a patient is too sick for surgery or cancer metastases are too far progressed.

For patients with extensive paralysis and advanced symptoms, the priority of care is dignity and comfort. Loss of bowel and bladder function can be distressing and lead to emotional withdrawal and skin breakdown.

Activity

Chapter 3 of the *Metastatic Spinal Cord Compression Full Guidance* document developed for NICE (National Collaborating Centre for Cancer 2008) explores the patient experience.

Consider the following narrative from this chapter by a patient's relative and list the care interventions needed to help support the patient and family:

On the 4th day he had surgery to stabilise the spine but sadly this was all done far too late as the damage was done and he was left with no use of his legs, trunk or right arm (National Collaborating Centre for Cancer 2008:16).

In particular, consider the impacts the following may have on both the patient and family:

- A delay in surgery.
- The loss of use of the right arm.
- What the underlying diagnosis might be.
- Lower limb paralysis.

Considering the impact on both the patient and family is part of the assessment process and is important in planning effective care.

NMC Domain 1: 1.4
NMC Domain 2: 2.3; 2.4; 2.5
NMC Domain 3: 3.7

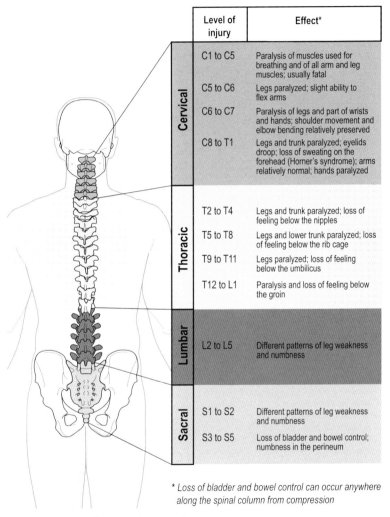

Level of injury		Effect*
Cervical	C1 to C5	Paralysis of muscles used for breathing and of all arm and leg muscles; usually fatal
	C5 to C6	Legs paralyzed; slight ability to flex arms
	C6 to C7	Paralysis of legs and part of wrists and hands; shoulder movement and elbow bending relatively preserved
	C8 to T1	Legs and trunk paralyzed; eyelids droop; loss of sweating on the forehead (Horner's syndrome); arms relatively normal; hands paralyzed
Thoracic	T2 to T4	Legs and trunk paralyzed; loss of feeling below the nipples
	T5 to T8	Legs and lower trunk paralyzed; loss of feeling below the rib cage
	T9 to T11	Legs paralyzed; loss of feeling below the umbilicus
	T12 to L1	Paralysis and loss of feeling below the groin
Lumbar	L2 to L5	Different patterns of leg weakness and numbness
Sacral	S1 to S2	Different patterns of leg weakness and numbness
	S3 to S5	Loss of bladder and bowel control; numbness in the perineum

* Loss of bladder and bowel control can occur anywhere along the spinal column from compression

Fig 15.7 Symptoms of spinal cord compression

Activity

The symptoms of MSSC can be diagnosed by a variety of assessment techniques.

Consider the role of the multiprofessional team in making a diagnosis. Make a list of how symptoms can be diagnosed by:

– direct observation

– conversation with a patient

– conversation with a family member

– medical tests.

To understand the role of the nurse in providing supportive measures for managing a patient with MSSC, read the article by Morgan and Cawley (2009) (see References).

NMC Domain 2: 2.1; 2.2; 2.3
NMC Domain 3: 3.1; 3.2

Hypercalcaemia

An increase in the normal amount of calcium in the blood is called hypercalcaemia. This is caused by cancer cells stimulating the release of calcium into the blood and involves osteoclast activity, bone resorption and the parathyroid gland. Normal blood calcium is between 2.2 mmol and 2.6 mmol. In a patient who has symptoms of hypercalcaemia, the blood calcium can be raised to over 3.5 mmol, and 3.75 mmol is an emergency situation which may lead to unconsciousness. For a patient with a cancer diagnosis, raised blood calcium is a sign of advancing disease and occurs in 10–20% of patients (Stewart 2005). Hypercalcaemia occurs more commonly in cancers of the breast, myeloma, lung, stomach, small intestine and prostate. Symptoms are associated with the rate of increase of calcium in the blood, rather than the actual amount of calcium. Commonly

a patient will experience nausea or/and vomiting, abdominal pain, dehydration, delirium and drowsiness. Sometimes a patient can get aggressive and this can be mistaken for terminal agitation. This is something we will look at in more detail in the Chapter 16.

Treatment is primarily by immediate rehydration using an intravenous infusion of normal saline over 24 hours. Once this is completed, medication called bisphoshonates will be started intravenously. The drugs used are either pamidronate or zolodronic acid. Bisphosphonates help to reduce bone resorption and lowered blood calcium can be seen after 2 to 3 days. Once a patient has had hypercalcaemia, they can have repeated episodes that can occur close together. Application of the ethical principles we looked at on page 47 must be applied when re-treating a patient.

Remember, it is always important to treat the person, not the blood result.

 Activity

Find out about the following terms:

■ Parathyroid hormone.

■ Bone resorption.

■ Osteoclasts.

For some of you, this may be physiology you have already studied during lecturers. If so, use this activity as a revision exercise. If it is new to you, look up each of the terms and make notes. Consider the link between the three terms and the impact this has on a patient. You might want to refer back to lecture notes or look at a core anatomy and physiology textbook to help consolidate your learning.

NMC Domain 1: 1.8
NMC Domain 3: 3.2
NMC Domain 4: 4.4

The principles of evaluating care

Another useful model in supporting patients with complex symptoms is the 'EEMMA' model (Twycross et al 2009). This is a more complex model than the three Cs model, providing a comprehensive way of assessing, planning, administering and evaluating care from the perspective of the whole team, and is used extensively in many specialist palliative care units.

The EEMMA model

- *Evaluation*: looking at a patient's story so far and includes considering what the cause of symptoms might be, the impact on the patient and what treatment has already been tried. Impeccable assessment is an essential part of the evaluation process.
- *Explanation*: considers what the patient and family understand about what is happening. Giving information and checking that the patient and family understand what is happening is an important part of ensuring they are fully involved in decision making.
- *Management*: this builds on the assessment process and looks at what symptoms are reversible. This is the first step and can be motivating to both the patient and family to see an improvement in symptoms, even if they are small.
- *Monitoring*: this is the responsibility of *all* team members. Noticing just a small change can have a big impact on the treatment plans. It is important to let patients know if there is a variety of treatment options available. This means that patients will not become disillusioned if medication or care intervention doesn't work as they know there are more options.
- *Attention*: keep showing an interest in the patient's story. It is always important to

 Activity

> Choose one of the symptoms you have been introduced to in this chapter that you would like to find out more about.
> Using the EEMMA model, make notes about how the symptoms can present and how the problems this brings for the patient can be managed in the clinical setting. Discuss the care management of this symptom with your mentor. Ask how different clinical areas might manage this symptom.
>
> NMC Domain 1: 1.1; 1.3
> NMC Domain 3: 3.1; 3.3

focus care on their experience of events and this avoids assumptions being made. Remember to avoid using jargon or making an assumption about the impact of symptoms on a patient's psychological wellbeing.

References

Ahlberg, K., Ekman, T., Gaston-Johansson, F., Mock, V., 2003. Assessment and management of cancer-related fatigue in adults. Lancet 363, 640–650.

Burzotta, L., Noble, H., 2010. Providing psychological support for adults living with cancer. End of Life Care 4 (4), 9–16.

Clancy, J., McVicar, A.J., 2009. Physiology and anatomy: a homeostatic approach, third ed. Hodder and Arnold, London.

Doyle, D., Hanks, G., Cherney, N., Calman, K., 2005. Oxford textbook of palliative medicine, 3rd ed. Oxford University Press, Oxford.

Drudge-Coates, L., Rajbabul, K., 2008a. Diagnosis and management of malignant spinal cord compression: part 1.

International Journal of Palliative Nursing 14 (3), 110–116.

Drudge-Coates, L., Rajbabul, K., 2008b. Diagnosis and management of malignant spinal cord compression: part 2. International Journal of Palliative Nursing 14 (4), 175–180.

Frith, H., Harcourt, D., Fussell, A., 2007. Anticipating an altered appearance: women undergoing chemotherapy for breast cancer. European Journal of Oncology Nursing 11 (5), 385–391.

Hinsley, R., Hughes, R., 2007. The reflections you get: an exploration of body image and cachexia. International Journal of Palliative Nursing 13 (2), 84–89.

Holdcroft, A., Power, I., 2003. Management of pain. British Medical Journal. 326, 635–639.

Holland, K., Jenkins, J., Solomon, J., Whittam, S. (Eds.), 2008. Applying the Roper–Logan–Tierney model in practice, 2nd ed. Churchill Livingston, Edinburgh.

International Association for the Study of Pain, 2007. Classification of chronic pain. Online. Available at: http://www.iasp-pain.org (accessed June 2011).

Levack, P., Graham, J., Collie, D., 2001. Don't wait for sensory level – listen to the symptoms: a prospective audit of the delays in diagnosis of malignant cord compression. Clinical Oncology 14, 472–480.

McCaffery, M., 1968. Nursing practice theories related to cognition, bodily pain and main environment interactions. University of California Student Store, Los Angles.

McCaffery, M., Pasero, C., 1999. Pain: clinical manual, 2nd ed. Mosby, St Louis.

Mock, V., Atkinson, A., Barsevick, A., et al., 2005. Cancer related fatigue. Clinical Practice Guidelines in Oncology. National Comprehensive Cancer Network, Fort Washington, PA.

Morgan, H., Cawley, D., 2009. Recognising metastatic spinal cord compression and treatment. End of Life Care 3 (4), 15–21.

National Collaborating Centre for Cancer, 2008. Metastatic spinal cord compression: diagnosis and management of patients at risk of or with metastatic spinal cord compression. Full guidance. National Institute for Health and Clinical Excellence, National Collaborating Centre for Cancer, London.

Nursing and Midwifery Council, 2008. The code: standards of conduct, performance and ethics for nurses and midwives. NMC, London.

O'Regan, P., Hegarty, J., 2009. Fatigue and depression in patients with advanced disease. End of Life Care 3 (2), 26–32.

Payne, S., Seymour, J., Ingleton, C., 2008. Palliative care nursing: principles and evidence for practice, 2nd ed. Open University Press, Maidenhead.

Piper, C., 2008. Assessment and management of the mouth at the end of life. End of Life Care 2 (1), 8–14.

Price, B., 2000. Altered body image: managing social encounters. International Journal of Palliative Nursing 6 (4), 179–185.

Ream, E., Richardson, A., 1996. Fatigue: a concept analysis. International Journal of Nursing Studies 33 (5), 519–529.

Roper, N., Logan, W., Tierney, A., 2000. The Roper–Logan–Tierney model of nursing: based on activities of living. Churchill Livingstone, Edinburgh.

Salter, M. (Ed.), 1997. Altered body image: the nurse's role. 2nd ed. Baillière Tindall, Edinburgh.

Stannard, S., 2008. Morphine: dispelling the myths and misconceptions. End of Life Care 2 (3), 7–12.

Stewart, A., 2005. Clinical practice: hypercalcaemia associated with cancer. New England Journal of Medicine 352, 373–379.

Stone, P., Richardson, A., Ream, E., et al., 2000. Cancer-related fatigue: inevitable, unimportant and untreatable? Results of a multi-centre patient survey. Annals of Oncology 119 (8), 971–975.

Twycross, R., Wilcock, A., Stark Toller, C., 2009. Symptom management in advanced cancer, 4th ed. palliativedrugs. com, Nottingham.

Uys, L., Habermann, M., 2005. The nursing process: globalisation of a nursing concept – an introduction. In: Habermann, M., Uys, L. (Eds.), The nursing process – a global concept. Churchill Livingstone, Edinburgh.

Websites

National End of Life Care Programme in England and Wales – gives details of best practice tools and national initiatives, http://www.endoflifecareforadults.nhs.uk/ (accessed November 2011).

East Midlands Cancer Network education site for the public and professionals. Contains news of local initiatives, practice guidelines on symptom management, communication and breaking bad/ significant news: http://www .eastmidlandscancernetwork.nhs.uk/ (accessed November 2011).

National Institute for Health and Clinical Excellence (NICE), Recommends evidence-based practice for a wide range of illnesses. There is a large section on cancer and cancer treatments offering guidance for clinicians: http://www.nice.org.uk (accessed November 2011).

16

Caring for patients at the end of life

CHAPTER AIMS

- To define end of life care
- To introduce the best practice tools used in end of life care
- How to recognise dying and managing the last days of life
- How to care for people from different faiths before and after death
- How to support bereaved relatives
- To explore how we can look after ourselves
- How to achieve national end of life care core competences

Introduction

Caring for a person at the end of life and offering support for their family and friends is a core part of nursing practice. You will potentially encounter end of life care in any clinical setting, of any age group and disease trajectory. This chapter explores the definitions associated with end of life care, and gives an overview of best practice tools and evidence base to care for a person before, at and after death. It presents individual exercises to support your developing knowledge across a variety of clinical placements. In these activities, you are encouraged to focus on your specific placement to help you put into practice your new knowledge, consolidate learning and provide evidence for NMC Competencies.

Definition of end of life care

End of life care is often associated with the last days of life. This chapter takes a wider view and considers end of life care as the last 'phase' of life. The National Council of Palliative Care (NCPC) suggests 'end of life care is simply acknowledged to be the provision of supportive and palliative care in response to the assessed needs of the patient and family during the last phase of life' (NCPC 2006a:3).

The *End of Life Care Strategy* builds on this working definition from the NCPC by outlining six keys steps needed to be considered as part of the patient's pathway (DH 2008:48):

1. Discussions as the end of life approaches.
2. Assessment, care planning and review.
3. Coordination of care for individual patients.
4. Delivery of high-quality services in different settings.

5. Care in last days of life.
6. Care after death.

Some parts of the county have developed these six key steps into a structured patient pathway that spans the last year of life. By having a structured pathway, it is possible to start to consider planning care in advance with the patient *and* their family, with the aim to limit decisions being made in a time of crisis. Figure 16.1 is an example of one of these pathways used within a health community in Nottinghamshire.

 Activity

Consider the pathway in Figure 16.1 and make notes about what challenges might be faced by the patient, family and care team in each of the phases:

- Last year of life.
- Last 6 months of life.
- Last weeks of life.
- Last days of life.
- After death.

Make a list of all the abbreviations you are not sure about and see if you can find out what they mean. Some are local to this specific health community and are included at the end of this chapter.

Now find out if your local health community has a specified pathway for last phase of life. It they do, how does it compare to the one in Figure 16.1?

NMC Domain 1: 1.4
NMC Domain 3: 3.3; 3.4; 3.5

The more definitive definition of end of life care used in the *End of Life Care Strategy* suggests it (DH 2008:47):

helps all those with advanced, progressive, incurable illness to live as well as possible until they die. It enables the supportive and palliative care needs of both patient and family to be indentified and met through the last phase of life and into bereavement. It includes management of pain and other symptoms and provision of psychological, social, spiritual and practical support.

Best practice tools in end of life care

In England, there are several tools that have been developed that are considered to be 'best practice' tools in end of life care. These tools have been widely distributed through the National End of Life Care Programme Website (http://www.endoflifecareforadults. nhs.uk/, accessed November 2011) and are advocated by the *End of Life Care Strategy* (DH 2008). We now look at each of these tools and consider how they might be used across a range of practice placements.

Liverpool Care Pathway (LCP)

This was developed by the Marie Curie Cancer Care charity at its hospice in Liverpool during the late 1990s. It was originally developed to support practitioners on acute wards at the local hospital, however it was recognised as a best practice tool in the NHS Beacon programme in 2001. Following this, it was included in the NHS End of Life Care programme in 2004. It is often referred to as the 'LCP'.

Initial assessment is by doctor and nursing teams and involves the patient and family taking a full and active part in communication. Information is given to relatives regarding facilities and support available, with consideration being made of faith, culture, values and beliefs. Symptoms are managed and unnecessary medication is stopped.

Ongoing assessment is then started and can be undertaken by any member of the

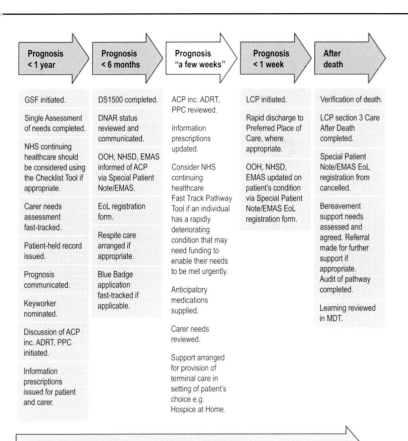

Fig 16.1 Last Year of Life Pathway (From Nottinghamshire End of Life Pathway for All Diagnoses (Next Stage Review Steering Group 2010). Reproduced with permission of NHS Nottingham City)

Table 16.1 Liverpool Care Pathway (adapted from version 12 of Liverpool Care Pathway)

Name: Mr Smith
NHS no: A123456
Date: 1.1.2010

Goal	04.00	08.00	12.00	16.00	20.00	24.00
(a) Patient does not have pain	A	A	V	A	A	A
(b) Patient is not agitated	A	A	V	A	A	A

team as appropriate. There are core goals of care to be achieved:

- The patient does not have pain.
- The patient is not agitated.
- The patient does not have respiratory tract secretions.
- The patent does not have nausea.
- The patient is not vomiting.
- The patient is not breathless.
- The patient does not have urinary problems.
- The patient does not have bowel problems.
- The patient does not have other symptoms. This can be a variety of things, for example an open wound needing dressing or a raised temperature.

This pathway offers guidance on achieving high-quality care in the last days of life as well as facilitating documentation of care that has been achieved. It is completed by all members of the care team and replaces medical, nursing and other uniprofessional notes, and becomes the central document of care for both the patient *and* the family.

The pathway is started when a patient is diagnosed as dying and focuses on goals to be achieved for high-quality last days of life care.

Four-hourly assessment of the patient and family will establish if a goal is achieved (A) or, if it is not achieved, this is referred to as a variance (V).

Looking at Mr Smith's written record in Table 16.1, we see he was pain free and not agitated at 08.00 since it is indicated that these two goals had been achieved (A). However, at 12.00, we see there were signs of a variance (V) away from goals (a) patient does not have pain and (b) patient is not agitated. This means Mr Smith was in some way displaying signs of both pain and agitation.

Any variance must be documented more fully on the 'variance analysis sheet', so we would expect to see something like the following written at 12.00:

Goal: (a) and (b)

Patient appears agitated and moaning. Gripping at bed sheets. Eyes rolling.

Given prn of levomepromazine and morphine as prescribed.

Signature: Staff Nurse Brown

Date/Time: 12.00 on 1.1.2010

Whenever a patient is recorded as having a variance (V), it is important to return soon afterwards to see if the care intervention has helped. So, for example, we might expect the next variance box to look something like this:

Goal: (a) and (b)

Mr Smith looks very settled and calm, face relaxed. Mrs Smith feels he in now much more settled.

Signature: Staff Nurse Brown

Date/Time: 12.25 on 1.1.2010

 Activity

Go to the Liverpool Care Pathway Website:

http://www.mcpcil.org.uk/liverpool-care-pathway/index.htm (accessed November 2011)

Familiarise yourself with the documentation and look at the patient-centred goals. Find out if the pathway is used in your practice placement. Your hospital or community setting might have an end of life pathway coordinator. If they do, find out if you can spend some time with them to see how they support practitioners with the use of the pathway.

NMC Domain 1: 1.1; 1.2; 1.3; 1.5; 1,6
NMC Domain 2: 2.7
NMC Domain 3: 3.1; 3.3

Gold Standards Framework

The Gold Standards Framework (GSF) was developed by Dr Kerri Thomas who, at the time, was a General Practitioner (GP) facilitator with Macmillan Cancer Relief. It was originally developed to assist GPs to work with the dying and their families, ensuring good symptom management was achieved. The framework includes the core themes of communication, coordination,

recognising dying and symptom management. Key parts of the framework are three triggers for supportive and palliative care:

1. The 'surprise question: would you be surprised if this patient died within a week? If yes, then consider: would you be surprised if this patient died in a month? Six months? A year? The answer to this question can help the team consider if the patient is in the last phase of life. While we might be surprised if a patient we are caring for dies in a week, we might not be surprised if they die in 6 months' time.
2. The patient with advanced disease makes a specific choice for comfort care only.
3. Clinical indicators of advanced disease are present: for example, increased agitation, falls, infections, pain and extreme fatigue. We look at these indictors later on in this chapter.

The GSF has now been introduced into care homes nationally and is currently being adapted for use in the acute hospital setting.

 Activity

Go to the National End of Life Care Programme Website and look up Gold Standards Framework:

http://www.endoflifecareforadults.nhs.uk (accessed November 2011)

Consider how it is used or can be introduced in your practice placement. Find out more about the term the 'surprise question'. Make some notes about the GSF and discuss it with your mentor. Ask if there are examples from your current placement where using the surprise question 'would you be surprised if' helped the care planning process.

NMC Domain 1: 1.1; 1.2
NMC Domain 3: 3.1; 3.3

Preferred Priorities of Care

Understanding what a patient wants is very important when providing holistic care. The Preferred Priorities of Care (PPC) document was originally developed by Marie Curie Cancer Care to help focus attention on what is a priority for the patient; what it is they want and hope for. It is now kept up to date by the Preferred Priorities of Care Review Team (2011) and this latest version is available from the National End of Life Care Programme Website. Very often you will see families speaking out for a patient. They mean well and may say 'He won't want to go into hospital' or 'He wouldn't want us upset by him dying in the house'. But how can we be sure this is what the patient wants? Instead, we need to be clear about what the patient wants, as well as understanding what is important to the family. Sometimes families can express their own fears and not the patient's wishes. So what they may be saying to you is 'I will feel so guilty if he goes into hospital' or 'How will we live in this house if he dies here'. The PPC contains various sections and supports patients in thinking though difficult issues and talking about the future.

 Activity

The following is a statement in the PPC 2011 document.
Include anything that is important to you or that you are worried about. It is a good idea to think about your beliefs and values, what you would and would not like, and where you would like to be cared for at the end of your life.

Consider how you may feel having a conversation with a patient focusing on this statement. Write down your worries or any specific skills you would like to develop while on this placement. Spend some time to formulate some key phrases that might be helpful when having a conversation about PCC. You can share these with you mentor to develop your confidence.

NMC Domain 1: 1.1
NMC Domain 3: 3.1; 3.3

Advance care planning

Planning ahead can help to avoid decisions being made in a crisis when a patient or family may be very distressed. An advance care plan (ACP) includes anything that helps towards having a plan that is clear to all those involved in the care of patients. It can include a PPC document, written notes about discussions with patients and families, a 'do not attempt cardiopulmonary resuscitation' (DNACPR) order and an 'advance decision to refuse treatment' (ADRT) order. Even a GP letter may contain details of what has been discussed with a patient and may include their future wishes.

Remember that it may be difficult to have some of these conversations with patients about refusing care, not being resuscitated and what they want their funeral to be like. But it can be far more distressing for the professional care team to work with families who are angry and distressed, where difficult conversations have not taken place or when a family is feeling they do not have any choices. Many of the conversations professionals can have with patients and family members will not require filling in a form. They are very important since they start to encourage individuals to think about their wishes and how they might communicate their choices, and are often referred to as general care planning.

The document *The Differences Between General Care Planning and Decisions Made in Advance* can be accessed through the National End of Life Care Programme Website and gives more detail about the concept of general and specific advance care planning:

http://www.endoflifecareforadults.nhs.uk/publications/differencesacpadrt (accessed November 2011)

Recognising dying and managing the last days of life

We have looked at some tools that can be used to help us care for the dying in their last phase of life. We now consider how we recognise dying in order to be able to use these tools. Recognising dying is not easy, even for the experienced professional (Furst & Doyle 2005). We must not take it for granted that other members of the team find this part of caring for a patient with advanced cancer simple and straightforward. Often the transition from curative cancer to last days of life care is complex. It can be a slow process or a sudden onset of new symptoms. Every patient must be assessed and treated individually. Patients tell us in many ways that they are dying. The challenge for the care team is to be aware of these signs to be able to recognise the dying.

 Activity

List the ways you might become aware that a person is dying.
What evidence did you use to identify these?

NMC Domain 1: 1.2
NMC Domain 2: 2.2; 2.3
NMC Domain 3: 3.1; 3.7; 3.10

There are some core signs and symptoms that are associated with dying. The NCPC suggests the commonly reported symptoms prior to death are increased pain or changes in the pattern of pain, restlessness and confusion, noisy breathing, nausea and vomiting, incontinence and extreme fatigue (NCPC 2006b). Furst and Doyle (2005) add falls, infections, unable to get out of bed and not wanting to eat or drink to this list. Some work done in long-term care homes in America asked the nursing staff how dying was recognised there with their residents (Porock & Oliver 2007). The core themes that emerged from these conversations with care home staff, described as 'patient cues', are: an adverse event, a decision, ready to go, withdrawal and the look. Let's see in detail what these five patient cues might look like in your practice placement.

An adverse event This can be falls happening or becoming more frequent, or recurring infections. These can happen for months prior to last days of life and are not always easy to link to end of life. This illustrates the importance of gathering information from relatives and getting the full story of what has happened in previous weeks and months. Sometimes family members can tell you 'They just haven't been right for months'. You might be involved in caring for a patient who is re-admitted with a fall or chest infection.

A decision Maybe this is to stop treatment or the patient starts to refuse fluids, food and medication. Conversations may change from the patient asking a lot of difficult questions, for example 'Am I dying?', to phrases like 'I know I am dying'

Being ready to go This might be changes in mood, or a patient might want to talk more about dying or sorting out their belongings. This is particularly challenging to manage when family members are not at the same stage or don't understand this change in behaviour.

Patient withdrawing The patient many no longer want to have certain visitors or stops talking with the patient in the next bed. Sometimes a patient may take down a photograph or not want to wash or prepare for visitors or not be interested in the news or sports results. This can be particularly distressing for family members, especially when they are actively involved in their care. Withdrawing can happen weeks or days prior to the death.

The look The patient may be pale with changes in skin colour which becomes mottled, a fall or rise in temperature, increasing agitation and changes to breathing patterns. You might return to your placement area after a few days off and notice a patient is looking more tired, or just very pale.

✋ Activity

Return to the list you made in the previous activity about how dying might be recognised. Consider the things in your list. Are there any surprises in the five 'patient cues'? Now reflect on a patient you may have cared for who was dying. Make notes of how their symptoms might link to the cues to help recognise dying. Take a moment to stop and consider how you are feeling. Remembering to look after yourself is an important part of delivering safe and effective patient care.

NMC Domain 1: 1.2
NMC Domain 2: 2.4; 2.5
NMC Domain 3: 3.3; 3.4

Now we have spent some time thinking about how we might recognise dying and how to use the best practice tools available to use, let's look at how to manage some common symptoms experienced in the last days of life. Understanding why these symptoms are happening and how to ease a person's distress can really help you feel confident when supporting a patient and family at this distressing time. Managing the last days of life can be both the most challenging parts of nursing care, yet also the most rewarding.

We now look at care in the last days and hours of life by specifically considering the challenging symptoms of terminal agitation and terminal secretions.

Terminal agitation

Restlessness, confusion and delirium are also terms associated with agitation in the last days and hours of life. We refer to terminal agitation, but the words and terms can be used interchangeably. It is important to understand why agitation occurs since 85% of patients with cancer will experience some degree of agitation, restlessness, delirium or confusion in the last weeks of their life (Macleod 1997). Biochemical changes that occur in the body as end of life approaches can affect the body's normal ability to filter and process stimulation and information received from the external environment, from within the body and from unconscious memories (Stedeford 1994). This means sensations and stimulation are not processed in the usual way and can become all muddled up, making it difficult for a patient to work out where the stimulation is coming from. For example, a simple noise may become frightening or a nurse call bell ringing may be interpreted as an alarm and may lead to a patient to try to get out of bed in fear. A full bladder might be interpreted as a memory from childhood leading the patient to call out for a deceased parent. A patient may be seen doing repetitive movements. To the patient these are purposeful, but for the family they can appear that the patient is distressed. Knowing about a person's life, work and hobbies can help to interpret these movements; a patient swinging both arms when lying flat may be playing golf, or circling the arms round each other may be winding wool.

Agitation may start as forgetfulness or changes in behaviour, mood or ability to speak words. It can often be a quick onset over just a few hours and sometimes more acute at night time with a complete reversal of sleep/wake patterns. You may see this if you work nights within your practice placement.

Accurate assessment of these changes is important by the whole care team and it is important to consider if there is anything that is reversible that might be causing the agitation. For example, a patient may be in withdrawal of nicotine if they have not been able to smoke a cigarette as they have deteriorated. Actions to reverse causes include replacing nicotine using patches, emptying the bladder, managing constipation or lowering a raised blood calcium level (Fig. 16.2). Once these have been tried, if the patient is still agitated it will probably mean that they are dying. It is always important to try to reduce anything that may be causing the agitation, even if this is the terminal phase, to reduce distress for the family. When caring for a patient with terminal agitation, it is important to keep stimulation in the environment to a minimum; encourage family members to read quietly at the bedside or bring in some favourite calming music to play softly.

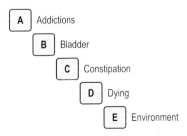

Fig 16.2 Checklist for terminal agitation.

Medication is also important and at this stage of a patient's life would be given subcutaneously. Particular care must be taken to managing the subcuataneous site since an agitated patient can easily dislodge a butterfly. Sometimes a subcutaneous site can become sore and this can be a source of distress, especially if it is in the upper arm and the patient is nursed on their side.

Terminal secretions

Noisy secretions occur in approximately 80% of patients at the end of life (Hughes et al 2000) and are often referred to as the 'death rattle'. This is more distressing for the relatives than the patient who, apart from having noisy breathing, can often be very settled and appear pain free. The secretions occur due to pooling of fluid in the pharynx which the patient does not have the energy to remove. This fluid can be saliva, produced as a result of an infection, pulmonary oedema or gastric reflux (Twycross et al 2009).

Nursing care is primarily to explain to the family why the secretions have occurred.

Repositioning the patient's head or lying them on their side with a pillow supporting their head can help to drain secretions. Occasionally, oropharyngeal suctioning can remove the secretions. Medication given subcutaneously needs to be started as soon as the secretions are noticed for it to be really effective. Hyoscine butylbromide or hysocine hydrobromide are the drugs of choice since they work as smooth muscle relaxants and have antisecretion effects. With good care, secretions can be reduced in half to one-third of patients in the last days of life. The choice of which of these drugs to use is reliant on local prescribing guidelines.

 Activity

Consider why the sound of secretions might be distressing to the family. Write out some sentences as to how you might explain this symptom. Being prepared and calm in responding to relatives' distress is really important so being prepared can help.

NMC Domain 1: 1.1; 1.3; 1.4
NMC Domain 2: 2.2; 2.3; 2.4
NMC Domain 3: 3.2

The care of people from different faiths before and after death

When a person dies in our care, it is the team's responsibility to ensure care and respect are shown not only to the relatives but also to the deceased person. Attention to spiritual, cultural and emotional issues is important. The care we give to the deceased is called 'last offices' and is the final act of care we can do to show our respect directly to our patient. Hospitals and community trusts will have specific guidelines on how to

perform these lasts offices. Generally, the care will include the following:

1. Finding out if there are any specific practices or rituals that are important for the patient and family.
2. First offices to ensure the deceased is clean and respectable for relatives who may want to visit immediately. This may include removing any unnecessary equipment from the bedside, washing the deceased's hands and face, brushing their hair, putting in dentures, etc.
3. Supporting relatives to see the deceased and say goodbye, recognising spiritual and religious needs.
4. Recording of the patient's property. Never remove jewellery without checking. If in doubt, leave it on ensuring it is accurately recorded before the deceased goes to the mortuary. Respect for property is important for relatives. Ensure it is folded and packed sensitively. Label all the bags with the deceased's name.
5. Last offices are prepared immediately before the deceased is transferred to the mortuary and includes full wash, being dressed in a white gown or clothing of the patients'/relatives' choice and takes into consideration infection control polices. When performing last offices, it is very important to be aware of cultural and spiritual practices important for the deceased and relatives.
6. Keeping relatives informed at all times of where the deceased is and when they are due to be transferred to the chapel of rest (mortuary).
7. Care of other patients needs to be timely and sensitive.

Remember that every patient and situation is different so you will be experiencing different emotions while undertaking similar duties. The care given to patients before, during and after death is call 'peri-death care'. One of the challenging areas of managing the last days of life, at death and after death is when the patient has

Activity

Imagine you are required to take part in last offices in your practice placement for a patient you have been looking after. How do you think you would feel? What specific worries do you think you may have? If this is something you have already taken part in, list the things that were difficult and the things that made doing this easier.

Now go and find the last offices guidelines for your practice placement. These are sometime called 'end of life guidance' or 'care after death'. Read through them and make a list of anything that you are not certain about or worried about. This can be used as part of your objective setting with your mentor. Find out what documentation needs to be completed and how the deceased is transported from your clinical placement to the mortuary and identify the roles of different colleagues who are involved in this process.

A useful document to support the care of the deceased is *Guidance for Staff Responsible for Care After Death (Last Offices)* which can be found on the National End of Life Care Programme Website:

http://www.endoflifecareforadults.nhs.uk/publications/guidance-for-staff-responsible-for-care-after-death (accessed November 2011)

NMC Domain 1: 1.1; 1.2; 1.5; 1.6
NMC Domain 2: 2.5; 2.7
NMC Domain 3: 3.4
NMC Domain 4: 4.4

a belief, culture or religion you are not familiar with. Being responsive to the needs and wishes of patients from other faiths and cultures means that you may sometimes be engaged in peri-death rituals that are new and unfamiliar to you.

Since religious and cultural beliefs can be a great source of strength at times of loss, it is helpful to understand what is meant by the terms 'culture' and 'ritual' in order to be able to appreciate the importance to groups of people.

We now look at the some terms individually.

Culture '... the values, norms and characteristics of a given group ... culture is one of the most distinctive properties of human social association ...' (Giddens 2009:1115). It is important to understand the strength culture has in the way a person behaves since, when a person comes into hospital, it is a meeting of their culture with

our own personal culture and then the professional culture of our organisation (Holland & Hogg 2010).

Values '... ideas held by human individuals or groups about what is desirable, good or bad ... what individuals value is strongly influenced by the specific culture in which they happen to live ...' (Giddens 2009:1136). Understanding the concept of values helps us with keeping our actions focused on what is important to the patient/family rather than our own perceptions of good and bad. This links to the ethical principles we explored in Chapter 5.

Religion '... a set of beliefs adhered to by members of a community involving symbols regarded with a sense of awe and wonder, together with ritual practices in which members of the community engage ...' (Giddens 2009:1130).

Table 16.2 Peri-death rituals in Hinduism

Before death	At death	After death
Sprinkled with Holy water	Sprinkled with Holy water	Tulsi leaf (basil) in mouth
Family present	Keep jewellery and threads	Postmortem allowed
Die near to mother earth	Close eyes and mouth	Cremation within 24 hours
Reciting of mantra/prayers	Mirrors covered	Women wear white
Lamp lit near the head	Loud wailing	Wrap in plain white cloth

Ritual '... essential to binding members of groups together ... they are found not only in regular situations of worship, but in various crises at which major social transitions are experienced ... birth, marriage and death ...' (Giddens 2009:531).

Understanding links between culture, religion and ritual are important when we are supporting a patient and their relatives. This awareness helps us to understand the important role commonly shared beliefs provide in terms of meaning and purpose (Giddens 2009) and is fundamental to meeting spiritual needs at times of distress.

Remember that care of a person's religious and cultural beliefs does not replace the care for their spiritual wellbeing. In Chapter 5, the definition of spirituality was introduced and an understanding of religion, culture and rituals helps to recognise spiritual needs.

As an example, we now explore some cultural aspects of a person who follows the Hindu religion. It is important to remember that not all Hindus will want the same thing or partake of the same rituals, just as people from different denominations within Christianity have different rituals and practices.

Hinduism is the world's oldest religion and has evolved over centuries, has its origins in the state of Gujerat, India, and believes in the worship of many Gods. Reincarnation and karma are sacred concepts meaning death is prepared for rather than feared.

Running water and cleanliness are very important to Hindus and a person who has died is seen as unclean, as are those who visit and care for them. Table 16.2 shows just a few of the rituals that are important in the Hindu faith. Don't forget that the patient, if well enough, and family are usually delighted to explain some of the rituals and beliefs. Don't be afraid to say to a family that you don't understand their rituals and practices. By asking, you are saying to them that it is important for you to know, therefore their beliefs and values are being respected too.

 Activity

Now go to the Ethnicity Online Website and look up a religion you are not familiar with, or continue to find out more about Hinduism:

http://www.ethnicityonline.net/ (accessed November 2011).

Click on 'ethnic/religious groups' and choose a group. You will then see that you have a choice to look up 'dying' and 'death and the dead'.

Read around pre- and post-death care for the religion you have chosen. Is there anything that confuses you? Are there any strange practices you would not feel comfortable being involved with? Consider why this might be. When you are in your practice placement, be prepared to consider if there are any rituals or practices you feel would be difficult to achieve and discuss these with your mentor.

For further reading to develop more awareness, you might want to look at the chapter 'Death and Bereavement: a Cross Cultural Perspective' by Holland in Holland and Hogg (2010) (see References). This chapter emphasises the importance of recognising culture and rituals in peri-death care. It is also particularly informative on the impact of culture on the bereavement process.

> NMC Domain 1: 1.2; 1.3
> NMC Domain 3: 3.3; 3.4
> NMC Domain 4: 4.4

role and often means sitting quietly with a family, passing on messages or making drinks. Find out how your clinical area supports the bereaved after they have left the ward. In some specialist areas, relatives can return a few days later to speak with staff.

 Activity

Consider your own feelings about supporting a bereaved family. This is something you may already have experience of. Take some time to think about what might be concerning you. Make a list of the things that might be important to the family.

> NMC Domain 1: 1.1; 1.5; 1.8
> NMC Domain 2: 2.5
> NMC Domain 3.4
> NMC Domain 4: 4.4

Supporting bereaved relatives

Even at times when a death is expected and has been prepared for by the care team, family members can become very distressed. Sometimes this is an expected part of their cultural beliefs in expression of grief and sometimes it can be unexpected. Thinking of somewhere that can offer privacy for a grieving family is helpful. Often relatives will want to ask about what to do next, where to get the certificate from and which funeral director to use. This can be a very confusing time where information is needed but not often remembered. Sometimes a practice placement will have leaflets that can be given to relatives to read when they get home. Familiarise yourself with these leaflets so you are able to refer to them if you are helping to support bereaved relatives. You may find that you are left with relatives when registered staff are busy. Being alongside a grieving person is an important

Looking after ourselves

The chapters you have worked through so far have provided you with a lot of information about cancer, treatment possibilities, dealing with difficult symptoms and managing the last phase of life. Much of this information may have been challenging for you. For some, it will be fairly straightforward, but others may be left with a lot of mixed emotions. Caring for yourself as you prepare for your practice placement, as well as looking after yourself while on placement, is vital. We now look at some ways you can care for yourself. The lessons you learn and tips for self-care can be taken with you into any part of your nursing career. Learning to care for yourself physically and emotionally while you are a student will put you in a good position to continue to care for yourself when qualified. It is also important to understand when a colleague may be emotionally struggling and know some ways to support them too.

Activity

For the next 6 days in a row, think of a treat for yourself, one each day. Rules about the treat:

■ It must not cost much money.

■ It must not take up too much time.

■ It must not contain too many calories!

Some example of treats: a house mate cooks your dinner; read a chapter of a novel when you get home from a placement or class; a special bubble bath only used as a treat; not answering the phone.

Being aware of when you are emotionally struggling is the first step in supporting yourself. This exercise can then be done to symbolically 'break the cycle' of feeling you do not have any time for yourself, so you can say to yourself 'I have treated myself' rather than 'I never have any time for me'. It is something you can take with you into the rest of your career. When you are working with colleagues who are stressed, it is something you can pass on to them to break their cycle too. Try it and then tell someone how you felt afterwards!

The following NHS Choices Website gives support and ideas to manage stress: http://www.nhs.uk/livewell/stressmanagement/Pages/Stressmanagementhome. aspx (accessed November 2011)

NMC Domain 1: 1.3; 1.7
NMC Domain 2: 2.5
NMC Domain 4: 4.4

National end of life care core competences

The End of Life Care Strategy (DH 2008) sets out clear guidelines for supporting the development of people working in health and social care who may be involved in a part of end of life care. These guidelines are called the *Core Competences for End of Life Care* (DH 2009) and are supported by a range of health and social care agencies. There are five overall themes in the core competences and seven principles underpinning end of life care.

The five themes in the core competences are the following:

1. Communication: engage effectively with patients/residents/families in discussions about death and dying.

2. Assessment and care planning: holistically assess, develop, implement and review a plan of care involving the family, patient or resident as appropriate.

3. Symptom management: provide quality symptom management with their level of competence and know when it is appropriate to refer to specialist palliative care.

4. Advance care planning: engage in advance care planning discussion with patients/families/residents and show awareness of legal and ethical issues surrounding the advance care planning process.

5. Overarching values and knowledge: demonstrate awareness of own values, knowledge and ongoing professional development in supporting people

experiencing loss, grief and bereavement from a variety of social, cultural and religious backgrounds.

The seven principles underpinning end of life care are the following:

1. Choices and priorities of the individual are at the centre of planning and delivery.
2. Effective, straightforward, sensitive and open communication between individuals, families, friends and workers underpins all planning and activity. Communication reflects an understanding of the significance of each individual's beliefs and needs.
3. Delivery through close multidisciplinary and interagency working.
4. Individuals, families and friends are well informed about the range of options and resources available to them to be involved with care planning.
5. Care is delivered in a sensitive, person-centred way, taking account of circumstances, wishes and priorities of the individual, family and friends.
6. Care and support are available to anyone affected by the end of life and death of an individual.
7. Workers are supported to develop knowledge, skills and attitudes. Workers take responsibility for, and recognise the importance of, their continuing professional development.

Some of these core competences have been introduced in previous chapters, and the principles underpin all the care that is planned and provided for a patient facing life's end. Employers from across health and social care will be looking for new employees who have these core competencies. Many employers have already included them as part of the annual professional development review for each employee.

Further information on the core competencies and levels to achieve across health and social care is available from the National End of Life Care Programme Website:

http://www.endoflifecareforadults.nhs.uk/publications/corecompetencesframework (accessed November 2011)

The final chapter of this section focuses on survival after a cancer diagnosis and treatment. Remember, having a cancer diagnosis does not mean a person will die. Let's now look at some positive statistics and what life is like living beyond cancer.

References

Department of Health, 2008. End of life care strategy: promoting high quality care for all adults at the end of life. Department of Health, London.

Department of Health, 2009. Core competences for end of life care. Department of Health, London.

Furst, C., Doyle, D., 2005. The terminal phase. In: Doyle, D., Hanks, G., Cherny, N., Calman, K. (Eds.), Oxford textbook of palliative medicine, 3rd ed. Oxford University Press, Oxford.

Giddens, A., 2009. Sociology, 6th ed. Polity, Cambridge.

Holland, K., Hogg, C., 2010. Cultural awareness in nursing and health care: an introductory text, 2nd ed. Edward Arnold, London.

Hughes, A., Wilcock, A., Corcoran, R., et al., 2000. Audit of three antimuscarine drugs for managing retained secretions. Palliative Medicine 14 (3), 221–222.

Macleod, A., 1997. The management of delirium in hospice practice. European Journal of Hospice Care 4 (4), 116–120.

National Council of Palliative Care, 2006a. End of life care strategy: the NCPC submission. NCPC, London.

National Council of Palliative Care, 2006b. Changing gear: guidelines for managing the last days of life in adults. NCPC, London.

Next Stage Review Steering Group, 2010. The Nottinghamshire end of life care pathway for all diagnoses, issue 2. Nottinghamshire.

Porock, D., Oliver, D., 2007. Recognizing dying by staff in long term care. Journal of Hospice and Palliative Nursing 9 (5), 270–278.

Preferred Priorities of Care Review Team, 2011. Preferred priorities for care. Online. Available at http://www.endoflifecareforadults.nhs.uk/assets/downloads/PPC_document_v22_rev_20111.pdf (accessed May 2011).

Stedeford, A., 1994. Facing death: patients, families and professionals. Sobell, Oxford.

Twycross, R., Wilcock, A., Stark Toller, C., 2009. Symptom management in advanced cancer, fourth ed. palliativedrugs.com, Nottingham.

Websites

National End of Life Care Programme guidance, http://www.endoflifecareforadults.nhs.uk/care-pathway/6-careafterdeath and http://www.endoflifecareforadults.nhs.uk/publications/pubacpguide (accessed November 2011).

General Medical Council guidance on treatment and care towards the end of life, http://www.endoflifecareforadults.nhs.uk/publications/gmceoltreatmentandcare (accessed November 2011).

Ethnicity Online details of peri-death rituals across a range of religions and cultures, http://www.ethnicityonline.net/ (accessed November 2011).

National Council for Palliative Care, http://www.ncpc.org.uk/ (accessed November 2011).

Marie Curie Cancer Care, http://www.mcpcil.org.uk/ (accessed November 2011).

NHS Choices Website offers guidance on assessment and management of stress, http://www.nhs.uk/livewell/stressmanagement/Pages/Stressmanagementhome.aspx.

Abbreviations

ACP, advance care plan.
ADRT, advance decision to refuse treatment.
BLUE BADGE, disability badge to display in car.
DNAR, do not attempt resuscitation.
DS1500, financial claim form.
EMAS, East Midlands Ambulance Service.
GSF, Gold Standards Framework.
OOH, Out of Hours (this service is often run by a combined group of GPs).
PPC, preferred priorities of care.

17 Living with and beyond cancer

CHAPTER AIMS

- To introduce the concept of survivorship
- To understand the transition from acute care and treatment into follow up
- To understand the potential long-term consequences of cancer and its treatment
- To appreciate the supportive strategies required by those living with and beyond cancer to live a healthy and active life.

Introduction

Once individuals with cancer have completed their treatment, they enter an uncertain time: Am I cured? Will it come back? What now? It is vital to understand that when cancer treatment ends, it doesn't mean the end of the 'cancer experience' for the patient. Patients who have had a cancer diagnosis experience multiple ongoing problems which require psychological, social and economic adjustment and self-management of altered physical functioning long after the completion of cancer treatment and they require long-term support.

Due to the older population being more susceptible to cancer, many patients with cancer have other co-morbidities and many of them will be admitted to acute clinical areas or be cared for in the community setting at some point in their life. For instance, they may be admitted for a non-cancer-related health issue such as cardiovascular disease or a respiratory problem or for a surgical procedure such as a hernia repair.

Therefore, it is highly likely you will meet and care for people who have had, or still have, a diagnosis of cancer on a variety of placements, as well as throughout your nursing career wherever you decide to work as a qualified nurse. So it is important that you understand what these individuals might have experienced and consider how they might still be affected, in order to provide support and care.

The general public frequently associate a diagnosis of cancer with death. In reality, the situation is often very different. Health policy in the UK has focused on prompt diagnosis and national equity of evidence-based treatment, resulting in earlier cancer detection and wider availability of effective cancer treatments, thus reducing the mortality rates (DH 1995, 1998, 2000,

2004). Consequently, the UK is experiencing increasing numbers of individuals surviving a cancer diagnosis and treatment (5-year survival = 56% for women, 43% for men; 10-year survival = 52% women and 39% men (Office for National Statistics (ONS) 2007)).

There are currently 1.6 million people living in England with a cancer diagnosis. This number is predicted to rise by over 3% per year (ONS 2008). By 2030, it is estimated that over 3 million people will be living with or beyond a cancer diagnosis in England (DH et al 2010). This increase has significant implications for individual patients and for the health service in terms of how this group of patients can best be managed and supported in the longer term.

Cancer is increasingly becoming a chronic disease, characterised by intense treatment, remissions and long periods of outpatient follow up (Dennison & Shute 2000). Once active treatment is complete and patients return home, contact with healthcare professionals diminishes and family members are increasingly required to contribute to the patients' physical and psychological management. This demanding role often results in physical and emotional repercussions for the lay carer (Badr & Carmack Taylor 2006).

Although many cancer survivors return to previous employment and lifestyles, attempting to put the cancer diagnosis and cancer treatment behind them, there is a higher incidence of chronic illness and disability in cancer survivors compared with those without a cancer diagnosis (Sugimura & Yang 2006). Patients may experience physical and psychosocial problems that result from the disease itself or its treatment. Some problems have a time limit, others persist, while others may not appear until months or years later (Cooley 2000). Currently, the long-term effects of cancer treatment are not systematically identified or recorded; there are few diagnostic or integrated care pathways linking changes in

health resulting from the consequences of cancer treatments and few specialist services are available for those with ongoing complex needs.

The concept of survivorship

So when does someone become a 'cancer survivor'? Traditionally we have thought of survivorship, in terms of the medical end point of treatment and when the patient is discharged from hospital follow-up care, at either 1 or 5 years. However, in reality, these time points are irrelevant to the patient and do not reflect the ongoing consequences of the disease and treatment. The National Coalition for Cancer Survivorship (1986) considers that an individual is a cancer survivor from the time of diagnosis, through the balance of his or her life. Family members, friends, and caregivers are also impacted by the survivorship experience and are therefore included in this definition. This definition highlights that it isn't just the patient who is affected by the consequences of cancer and its treatment, and that these consequences commence from the time of symptom presentation or diagnosis and continue throughout the duration of an individual's life. Mullan (1985) proposes that survivorship is transitional, rather than a series of distinct stages, and there are three phases of survival: *acute* (during the diagnostic phase); *extended* (when treatment is over); and *permanent* survival. To date, there has been a lack of attention given to the *extended phase* of post-treatment and very little exploration of what are the best strategies to support these patients through the transition of these phases.

Much of the literature and research has been completed in the USA and is referred to as 'survivorship'. Patients in the UK tend to dislike this label, as it implies victim status. For this reason, the phrase 'living with and beyond cancer' has be adopted (Macmillan Cancer Support 2008a, DH et al 2010).

The transition from acute care and treatment into follow up

Patients often experience negative emotions towards the often abrupt withdrawal of intensive support (from healthcare professionals, family and friends) once treatment is complete. This is often associated with ambivalence to discontinuation of treatment, signifying the loss of a security blanket (Moore 2011). Paradoxically, the post-treatment period is idealised by family and friends who attempt to persuade the individual they are lucky and encourage them to 'get back to normal'. Although patients convey a need to resume life, there is recognition and frustration that life before cancer cannot be resumed and patients and carers may feel confused when feelings of anxiety and depression linger after the patient has been told treatment has been successful. Rather than 'getting back to normal', patients need to adjust to a new situation and, although the cancer may have physically been removed, the effects of cancer and treatment as well as feelings accompanying the experience may not leave them.

The end of treatment is associated with a number of transitions for patients and their families as they shift from the 'long haul' of active treatment to a state of limbo. Without the continual hospital visits, an individual may have more time and opportunity to reflect on what has happened to them and contemplate what the future may hold. They may start to ask questions such as: What are my chances of having children? Should my family be tested? Will the cancer come back? Why don't I feel in control? What happens now?

Once treatment has been completed, patients will be seen in an outpatient setting for a 'follow-up' appointment. The purpose of this is to review the patient's physical health and assess the response to treatment. However, the value and purpose of formal follow-up clinic appointments in relation to the management of cancer patients has been debated over the past few decades. Rather than a means of support or providing information, traditionally the emphasis of follow-up appointments has been focused on record keeping, disease surveillance, detection and treatment of recurrence (Torjesen 2010). However, the effectiveness and efficiency of follow-up to detect recurrent cancer has been disputed (Alberts 2007).

Activity

Talk to a patient who is coming to the end of their treatment. Find out how they will be followed up by the healthcare team. Find out how the patient feels about this.

NMC Domain 1: 1.3; 1.4
NMC Domain 2: 2.4; 2.5
NMC Domain 3: 3.5

Alongside this, the health system is under enormous pressure to ensure people with a suspected cancer are seen by a specialist within a 2-week target of being referred by their GP and patients diagnosed with cancer are treated within 31 days from diagnosis (DH 2004). This has increased the pressure on outpatient follow-up clinics and the appointment time between completing acute treatment and follow up for patients with cancer has lengthened. This affects the support and access to information and reduces the opportunities for patients and carers to ask questions.

Patients report mixed feelings regarding follow-up appointments: it may provide feelings of security and reassurance; reduce physical distress and anxiety; and is a way of providing information regarding prognosis and recovery. Conversely, many patients experience acute anxiety preceding follow-up appointments as they are confronted with fear of recurrence and a reminder of their experience. Often the focus of follow up is on the physical symptoms, largely ignoring psychosocial aspects (Torjesen 2010). It is also argued that due to regimented scheduling, the timing of follow-up appointments rarely coincides with patients experiencing anxiety and the need for questions to be answered. Patients often feel unable to contact healthcare professionals for information in between appointments or don't know who to ask for help.

Follow-up appointments are set in busy hospital clinics and are of a short duration, limiting the time available for patients to express concerns or seek information regarding rehabilitation and recurrence, and therefore are unlikely to provide the level of reassurance and support that patients need. Follow up could be initiated by the patient and should be driven by an assessment of the patient's need for support, rather than stipulated by protocol (Torjesen 2010). Patients may benefit from a 'debrief' by the treatment team at 1 and 6 months after the completion of treatment to discuss and clarify what happened (Johansson et al 1992). Telephone follow up has been shown to be acceptable and more convenient to patients. Phone calls are prearranged and made by a nurse specialist to find out about patients' progress and answer any questions they may have (Cox & Wilson 2003). These options are currently being explored by the National Cancer Survivorship Initiative task force (DH et al 2010). This is discussed later.

 Activity

Find out how patients are followed up in the short and longer term in your placement area once they have completed their cancer treatment. Find out if there are any differences in how follow-up care is arranged and/or

delivered depending on the type of cancer a patient has. For instance, compare a patient who has had a head and neck cancer diagnosis and a patient with a breast cancer diagnosis. Are there differences in the frequency of appointments and the duration of follow-up care before the patient is discharged completely? Why might these variations exist?

NMC Domain: 1.3; 1.5; 1.6
NMC Domain 3: 3.3; 3.8
NMC Domain 4: 4.6; 4.7

The potential long-term consequences of cancer and its treatment

Physical impact

Historically, the long-term consequences of cancer and its treatment have been difficult to research, due to the high mortality rates associated with the disease. The extent of physical impact will depend on the type of cancer; types and combination of treatments given; pretreatment performance status; presence of co-morbidity; and prompt recognition and intervention of toxicities. These will influence the long-term health and quality of life among survivors. Although the severity of symptoms may diminish over time, debilitating symptoms such as pain, fatigue, poor appetite, weight loss, insomnia, loss of fertility, hormone alteration and impaired sexual functioning can persist for many months/years, associated with a poor quality of life (Brant et al 2011). For example, the extent of surgery will vary depending on whether the patient is undergoing curative treatment and whether they are physically well enough to undergo the procedure.

The more extensive the surgery, the more physically compromised a patient will be postoperatively.

The Macmillan health and wellbeing survey (Macmillan Cancer Support 2008b) identified that 78% of patients living beyond cancer experience at least one physical health problem within 12 months of completing treatment and 71% of patients who finished treatment 10 years ago continue to experience physical health problems. To give a specific illustration of this, 21% of patients spend most of the day in bed due to respiratory problems 12 months following the surgical removal of lung cancer (Sarna et al 2004); 30% of patients with lung cancer express significant chronic pain 4 years postoperatively (Karmaker & Ho 2004) and almost all patients report debilitating shortness of breath 10 years after surgery affecting their quality of life and requiring long-term adaptation (Maliski et al 2003).

Activity

Identify a patient you are caring for. Using their medical/nursing notes, list the treatments they have had so far, look up the long-term side effects and consider how the patient might be physically affected by this.

NMC Domain 1: 1.7; 1.9
NMC Domain 3: 3.4; 3.8; 3.9

Psychosocial impact

Unsurprisingly, the burden of physical symptoms experienced by patients recovering from cancer treatments has a significant long,term impact on psychosocial wellbeing, as well as affecting the emotional wellbeing of spouses (Sarna & McCorkle 1996). The majority of cancer patients experience uncertainty, anxiety, apprehension, loss of confidence, loss of normality, lower sexual activity and have unrealised employment and retirement plans due to the physical limitations of treatment and disease. Yet healthcare professionals generally underestimate psychological symptoms. For example, 66% of patients with lung cancer report anxiety as a significant problem, yet healthcare professionals estimate only 23% of patients with lung cancer experience anxiety; 49% of patients report depression but consultants do not recognise this at all (Krishnasamy et al 2001). Many patients meet and become friends with other patients. This can be a great source of support, however it may be quite distressing if another patient dies. As well as heightening the sense of their own mortality, they may feel a sense of guilt: 'Why wasn't it me?'

Uncertainty is a significant issue for the majority of patients and their family members as there are many questions that cannot be answered: What will the outcome of treatment be? Has the cancer gone completely? What will the long-term outcome be? The fear of recurrence is an emotional burden to a greater or lesser extent for the majority of patients and carers (Llewellyn et al 2008). Often referred to as the 'Sword of Damocles' which hangs over the individual and family for the rest of the person's life, the fear of recurrence creates anxiety and uncertainty for the future, as well as interfering with normal daily living. This fear may diminish over time or may continue to be a long-term problem (Ronson & Body 2002).

Many patients feel concerned that they will not know what signs and symptoms to look for, especially if they did not have any symptoms at the time of diagnosis, or fear that they will not recognise any signs or symptoms. A routine cough or pins and needles can cause worry and distress by assuming that the cancer has returned. At the same time, people may not want to bother healthcare professionals as 'It is probably nothing' or they are unsure who they should tell – the GP or the oncologist?

Conversely, a cancer diagnosis may trigger a greater appreciation of life (Wyatt et al 1993). Once treatment has finished, some individuals take stock and reprioritise their plans and life objectives, making more time for important activities. There may be changes in lifestyle behaviours, such as eating habits and other healthy activities.

There are many long-lasting visible reminders of the events and experiences of cancer, such as postoperative scars, scars from where a central venous access device has been removed, discoloration of the skin or a change of bodily functioning. However small these may be, they may alter an individual's perceived body image and may affect confidence, relationships, employment, leisure activities, etc. Diminished physical functioning may impact on an individual's ability to fullfil their social role as a parent, partner, child, sibling, etc. which may have a dramatic impact on family and social situation. They may not be able to return to their original place of work or resume leisure activities, which in turn affects perception of quality of life as well as financial stability.

 Activity

> Think about the patient you identified earlier in this chapter. What might the long-term psychosocial impact be?
>
> Watch the Institute of Medicine 'Lost in transition' video on YouTube:
>
> http://www.youtube.com/watch?v=YhuqWM3dNAw (accessed November 2011)
>
> NMC Domain 2: 2.4
> NMC Domain 3: 3.1; 3.3; 3.4

Economic and employment impact

Depending on the nature of employment and the type/severity of cancer and treatment-related side effects, many patients attempt to continue to try to retain their role and routine, as well as maintain an income, while undergoing treatment. Many people do not have employment sick pay or leave schemes, so if they do not work they do not get paid. Many continue to work as they fear that they will lose their job, due to the numerous absences to attend hospital appointments and receive treatments, and time off to recover from the consequences of toxicities. Being a patient can also be very costly with multiple prescriptions, car parking, etc. Unsurprisingly, 92% of people affected by cancer suffer loss of income and/or higher costs. Patients under 55 years old suffer an average fall in income of 50%, causing significant hardship (RDSi research commissioned by Macmillan Cancer Relief 2006).

Even if patients return to work after treatment, they may feel trapped in their job or feel that their options for promotion are limited. They may not feel able to move to a new employer, in case of risking loss of sick pay/leave. It may be more difficult to secure a new position if an occupational health screen is required. They may face the dilemma of whether they should tell their potential employer at all about their diagnosis. In 2005, the Disability Discrimination Act was extended to apply to cancer patients from the point of diagnosis. The Act gives individuals who have/had a cancer diagnosis protection from discrimination in employment and education. However, only one in five employers are aware that cancer is covered by the Act. This makes patients very vulnerable to losing their jobs and they themselves often do not realise that they are protected by the Act (Simm et al 2007). The Equality Act (2010) replaces current discrimination laws, including the Disability Discrimination Act (1995), bringing them all together under one piece of legislation. The Act aims to make discrimination legislation more consistent, clearer and easier to follow.

As well as the issues of employment, patients experience a number of other financial challenges. For instance, once diagnosed with cancer, it is increasingly difficult to get a mortgage, financial loan, travel and life insurance. Insurance premiums are significantly higher than before diagnosis.

The supportive strategies required by those living with and beyond cancer to live a healthy and active life

In order for patients and family members to adjust, they need to understand their situation and identify coping strategies to self-manage the functional, socioeconomic and emotional consequences of cancer and its treatment.

Healthcare professionals need to look beyond acute treatment and provide support and information outlining what to expect in terms of late side effects; how long these symptoms might persist; what rehabilitation services and strategies are recommended; what benefits they are entitled to; what signs and symptoms of recurrence to look for; and, overall, who, when and where to seek advice from.

More challenging is how to manage the *unanswerable* questions such as 'Am I cured?' and 'Will it come back?' Llewellyn et al (2008) suggest that it is impossible to eliminate uncertainty and fear of recurrence, but by developing patients' cancer knowledge, they can manage using emotional and problem-based coping strategies. This suggests the need to evaluate the current focus of health care and a shift in attitudes and approaches is required to support individuals beyond cancer treatment. All healthcare interventions should have the long-term interest of patients as the focus point (Doyle 2008).

To date, there has been little policy recognition of the concept of survivorship or how best to support patients beyond the acute phase of treatment. *The Cancer Reform Strategy* (DH 2007) is the first policy setting out a commitment to improve patients' experience of living with and beyond cancer. From this report, the National Cancer Survivorship Initiative (NCSI) was established. The NCSI vision (DH et al 2010) sets out to determine the possible approaches to survivorship care and how these can best be tailored to meet individual patients' needs. This work focuses on creating long-term holistic assessment and care planning, ensuring that post-treatment care is practical and sustained. A single record of treatment is proposed, written intelligibly for patients outlining the basis of conversations about their care and a summary of the type of cancer; what procedure/treatment they had received; what to expect immediately post-treatment; what the consequences of treatment might be in the medium to long term; what patients can do optimise their recuperation and recovery; how long side effects and symptoms may last; what signs and symptoms of recurrence to watch for; and how they would be followed up.

There remain significant discrepancies between the ideas of patients, GPs and oncologists of which healthcare professional should follow patients up. Some patients desire follow-up care with their consultant (Cheung et al 2009). However, many patients are not seen by the consultant in follow-up care. Other patients prefer to be followed up by their GP as they know their case more thoroughly than anyone and the patient has easier access to them. However, patients perceive that the GP may not actually possess the in-depth specialist knowledge and skill to provide care. A GP 'review and recall system' is also proposed, ensuring appropriate, patient-specific, primary care for cancer survivors. GPs perceive themselves to have a central role in follow up, disease surveillance and screening for other cancers (Cheung et al 2009).

However, currently no healthcare professional role facilitates self-management by empowering and enabling patients and carers to identify resources and skills to self-manage. Medical roles focus on cure and managing the immediate effects of treatment and disease surveillance. There are very few community-based rehabilitation services.

The NCSI proposes the role of a dedicated key worker, who could work in partnership with individual patients, assessing and identifying their needs from diagnosis through to follow up, and collaborate and communicate across all service providers (not necessarily based at the hospital) as a central coordinator, directing patients to other specialist healthcare professionals. However, this would be logistically challenging within the current infrastructure and financial situation of the NHS, and considerable research, redirection of resources and redesign would be required.

Nevertheless, a new model of transitional care is required to ensure that acute and primary care services effectively manage and provide long-term, consistent, reliable care based on individual need. As healthcare professionals, we have a responsibility to provide information and support to individuals living with and beyond cancer to enable them to self-manage the significant physical, socioeconomic and emotional effects of the disease and it treatment, as wells as adopt healthy lifestyle behaviours.

References

Alberts, W.M., 2007. Follow up and surveillance of the patient with lung cancer: what do you do after surgery? Respirology 12, 16–21.

Badr, H., Carmack Taylor, C.L., 2006. Social constraints and spousal communication in lung cancer. Psychooncology 15, 673–683.

Brant, J.M., Beck, S., Dudley, W.N., et al., 2011. Symptom trajectories in post treatment cancer survivors. Cancer Nursing 34 (1), 67–77.

Cheung, W.Y., Neville, B.A., Cameron, D.B., et al., 2009. Comparison of patient and physician experience for cancer survivorship care. Journal of Clinical Oncology 27, 1.

Cooley, M.E., 2000. Symptoms in adults with lung cancer: a systemic research review. J. Pain. Symptom. Manage. 19 (2), 137–153.

Cox, K., Wilson, E., 2003. Follow-up for people with cancer: nurse led services and telephone interventions. Journal of Advanced Nursing 43 (1), 51–61.

Dennison, S., Shute, T., 2000. Identifying patients concerns: improving the quality of patient visits to the oncology out-patient department – a pilot study. European Journal of Oncology Nursing 4, 91–98.

Department of Health, 1995. A policy framework for commissioning cancer services. Calman-Hine report). HMSO, London.

Department of Health, 1998. A first class service: quality in the new NHS. HMSO, London.

Department of Health, 2000. The NHS cancer plan. HMSO, London.

Department of Health, 2004. The NHS cancer plan and the new NHS. HMSO, London.

Department of Health, 2007. The cancer reform strategy. HMSO, London.

Department of Health, Macmillan Cancer Support and NHS Improvements, 2010. National Cancer Survivorship Initiative: vision. HMSO, London.

Doyle, N., 2008. Cancer survivorship: evolutionary concept analysis. Journal of Advanced Nursing 62 (4), 499–509.

Johansson, S., Steinbeck, G., Hursti, T., et al., 1992. Aspects of patient care. Interviews with relapse free testicular patients in Stockholm. Cancer Nursing 15, 54–60.

Karmaker, M.K., Ho, A.M., 2004. Post thoracotomy pain syndrome. Thoracic Surgery Clinics 14, 345–352.

Krishnasamy, M., Wilkie, E., Haviland, J., 2001. Lung cancer health care needs assessment: patients' and informal carers' responses to a national mail questionnaire survey. Palliative Medicine 15, 213–227.

Llewellyn, C.D., Weinman, J., McGurk, M., Humphris, G., 2008. Can we predict which head and neck survivors develop a fear of recurrence? Journal of Psychosomatic Research 65, 525–532.

Macmillan Cancer Support, 2008a. Two million reasons: the cancer survivorship agenda. Macmillan Cancer Support, London.

Macmillan Cancer Support, 2008b. Health and wellbeing survey. Macmillan Cancer Support, London.

Maliski, S.L., Sarna, L., Evangelista, L., Padilla, G., 2003. The aftermath of lung cancer. Cancer Nursing 26 (3), 237–244.

Moore, A., 2011. Health and wellbeing clinics. A way out of limbo. The Health Service Journal Supplement 120 (6199), S4–S5.

Mullan, F., 1985. Seasons of survival: reflections of a physician with cancer. New England Journal of Medicine 313, 270–273.

National Coalition for Cancer Survivorship, 1986. Our history. Online. Available at: http://www.canceradvocacy.org/about-us/our-history.html (accessed November 2011).

Office for National Statistics, 2007. Mortality statistics: cause, 2005. ONS, London.

Office for National Statistics, 2008. Cancer statistics registrations. England, Series MB1, No. 37. Online. Available at: http://www.ons.gov.uk/ons/publications/index.html.

RDSi research commissioned by Macmillan Cancer Relief, 2006. UK patient survey. (Unpublished).

Ronson, A., Body, J.J., 2002. Psychosocial rehabilitation of cancer patients after curative therapy. Support. Care Cancer 10, 281–291.

Sarna, L., McCorkle, R., 1996. Burden of care and lung cancer. Cancer Practice 4, 245–251.

Sarna, L., Evangelista, L., Tashkin, D., et al., 2004. Impact of respiratory symptoms and pulmonary function on quality of life of long term survivors of non-small cell lung cancer. Chest 125, 439–445.

Simm, C., Aston, J., Williams, C., et al., 2007. Organisations' responses to the Disability Discrimination Act. Report 410. Department for Work and Pensions, London.

Sugimura, H., Yang, P., 2006. Long-term survivorship in lung cancer – a review. Chest 129, 1088–1097.

Torjesen, I., 2010. A new approach to aftercare. The Health Service Journal Supplement 120 (6199), S2–S3.

Wyatt, G., Kurtz, M.E., Liken, M., 1993. Breast cancer survivors: an exploration of quality of life issues. Cancer Nursing 16 (6), 440–448.

Further reading

Cooley, C., 2010. Cancer survivorship, part 1: how services need to change for those living with and beyond cancer. Nursing Times 106 (20), 24–25.

Cooley, C., 2010. Cancer survivorship, part 2: providing advice and support to those living with and beyond cancer. Nurs. Times 106 (21), 17–18.

Davies, N.J., 2009. Cancer survivorship: living with or beyond cancer. Cancer Nursing Practice 8 (7), 29.

Ganz, P.A., 2011. The 3 'Ps' of cancer survivorship. BMC Med. 9 (14), 1–3.

McBride, S., Whyte, F., 1998. Survivorship and the cancer follow up clinic. European Journal of Cancer Care (Engl.) 7, 47–55.

Websites

National Cancer Survivorship Initiative, http://www.ncsi.org.uk/.

US National Coalition for Cancer Survivorship, http://www.canceradvocacy.org/.

World Cancer Research Fund (recommendations for cancer survivors to prevent cancer), http://www.wcrf-uk.org/cancer_prevention/recommendations/prevention_for_survivors.php.

Section 3. Consolidating learning: the patient experience

In this final section, you are encouraged to consolidate your learning by linking theory with experiences of cancer pathways from your practice placement. Making sense of these experiences can help ensure you move on to the next part of your training feeling motivated and confident, as well as gathering evidence for your NMC standards of competence. It is important to remember you will regularly be caring for people and family members from across all four fields of practice. For example:

- communicating with a relative who has a learning disability
- nursing a dying person who has a mental health diagnosis
- supporting a teenager with the decision-making process.

It is therefore important for you to consider how the competencies you have developed on this placement can be transferred to other clinical areas and care pathways.

In this section, learning is consolidated in two ways, first by putting the easy to use Driscoll model of reflection into practice. Second, a single case study explores the impact of diagnosis, the management of a range of side effects that may result from receiving cancer treatment and symptoms that may result from advancing disease. The case study then explores two parallel pathways that are a potential for this patient; end of life care or living beyond cancer. This facilitates you in applying theory to practice using a problem-solving approach across a cancer pathway. The final chapter helps to focus this consolidated learning by focusing on core nursing skills and action planning for future practice.

18 Introduction to consolidating learning

CHAPTER AIMS

- To introduce an easy to use model of reflection
- To link experiences and learning: learning to learn

An easy to use model of reflection

Making links between practical experiences, feelings and theory is an important part of the learning process and can result in enhancing professional practice over many years. An ideal way to make these links it to spend some time to reflect on your experiences, taking notice of the associated feelings and what these mean for you.

In Section 1, you were introduced to the Driscoll (2007) model of reflection (see appendix 1) which we use in this chapter to reflect on a variety of experiences from your practice placement.

First, refresh your knowledge on the Driscoll model:

- What? – returning to the situation.
- So what? – understanding the feelings.
- Now what? – thinking about what this means to you.

 Activity

Read the article by Burzotta and Noble (2011) (see References).

This is an excellent example of a reflection of interprofessional practice caring for a lady with advanced breast cancer using Gibbs model of reflection. Use this example to help you to develop you own reflections.

You may prefer to use a model of reflection you are familiar with or has been identified by your training school to do these exercises. Getting practice to use a specific model will help you gain the confidence to continue to use it throughout your future practice. Another way of reflecting on practice is to write freely about a situation. This is called a 'narrative approach' and is explored further in the work of Bolton (2010) (see References).

NMC Domain 1: 1.6; 1.7; 1.9
NMC Domain 3: 3.10
NMC Domain 4: 4.2; 4.7

Reflection point

Think of an experience that you found challenging on your placement. Make notes about this experience under each of the headings in the model. Now stop to consider how you are feeling about going back to this experience. Does it feel the same now as it did at the time? Think why this might be.

NMC Domain 1: 1.7; 1.8

Starting to understand why a certain situation may be challenging is an important step in ensuring you can respond effectively in the clinical environment. For example, a situation might be challenging because it has reminded you of a family situation, or because you did not feel supported by the staff you were working with or because you did not feel competent in performing a new skill. Once you can understand the feelings, you will be able to consolidate your actions for the next time you come across a similar situation.

Reflection point

Now think of an experience you found distressing to deal with or be part of. Make notes about this experience under each of the headings in the model.

Now stop to consider how you are feeling about going back to this experience. Does it feel the same now as it did at the time? Think why this might be.

Now consider what makes one experience feel challenging and another distressing.

NMC Domain 1: 1.7; 1.8

Recognising a range of feelings is important. Being able to separate out the situation from the feelings is an essential

part of developing to be a skilled practitioner. For example, a distressing situation might be supporting a family who are distressed when someone is dying. When reflecting back on this situation, you might find that while the situation was distressing, the associated feelings were really positive, since:
– you felt calm when supporting the relatives
– you were thanked by the relatives as they left the ward
– a team colleague who worked with you gave you positive feedback about achieving a competency
– you felt valued as a team member.
When you look to the third part of the model, what the experience means to you, the answer may be linked to:
– successfully achieving a level of competence/essential skill
– going to the next placement feeling more confident to do a specific task.

Linking experiences and learning: learning to learn

We now take some time to reflect on your experiences within the practice placement. This gives you the opportunity to explore what you have experienced and start to make sense of some of the things that you might have learnt, linking theory to practice. It is essential that you consider your placement experiences alongside the theory you have acquired in school and critically analyse and evaluate the clinical experience, to ensure both your own and other healthcare professionals' practice reflects contemporary research-based evidence.

This also gives you the chance to reflect on how you learn and what process works well for you to ensure you take positive strategies into your future practice. You are encouraged to refer back to Sections 1 and 2 to find answers to questions and to think using a problem-solving approach.

Making sense of experiences is crucial to your own developing professional practice. Learning from events, whether they are positive, challenging or disappointing, is a key step in being able to develop as a skilled and confident practitioner.

Having reflected on your experiences, you should have a good idea of where you are as a practitioner, enabling you to make an action plan of your future professional development. This process should not cease once you are qualified; you should continually and regularly take time to reflect on your experiences throughout your career, allowing you to keep abreast of changes in health care and to improve your professional performance.

References

Bolton, G., 2010. Reflective practice: writing and professional development, 3rd ed. Sage, London.

Burzotta, L., Noble, H., 2011. The dimensions of interprofessional practice. British Journal of Nursing 20 (5), 310–315.

Driscoll, J., 2007. Practising clinical supervision, 2nd ed. Baillière Tindall, Edinburgh.

Further reading

Bulman, C., Schutz, S., 2008. Reflective practice in nursing, 4th ed. Wiley-Blackwell, Oxford.

Website

Making Practic Based Learning Work project, http://www.science.ulster.ac.uk/nursing/mentorship/docs/learning/reflectiononpractice.pdf (accessed November 2011).

19   Introducing the case study

Chapters 19–24 follow a patient diagnosed with breast cancer, in the form of a case study. Each chapter identifies a stage of the patient experience. As the case study unfolds, there are a number of activities to complete. In each activity, you are given the opportunity to explore a variety of nursing interventions and provide holistic support for both the patient and her family. You are encouraged to refer back to the anatomy and physiology, and other health theory, in Sections 1 and 2. Practical exercises are suggested for you to do either while on placement or by reflecting on previous experience. It is, therefore, useful to have your notes from Sections 1 and 2 handy since you will be directed back to some of the activities you have already completed.

By working through one patient experience in this way, you can follow through aspects of integrated care introduced throughout the book. You are also encouraged to link the NMC principles and competencies to various stages of the patient's experience.

Journal papers are suggested for each of the exercises. These papers may not refer specifically to the cancer experience, but encourage you to think across different disease groups. For example, section on complex discharge suggests a paper exploring the challenges of discharging a woman with multiple sclerosis. This helps

to focus and consolidate and build up your knowledge, as well as provide underpinning evidence to apply confidently in your future clinical practice across a range of clinical settings.

From the point of diagnosis, patients encounter many different physical, psychological, social and economical effects of cancer and its treatment. Their experience will be unique and the time frame for each individual will be different. As healthcare professionals, we are generally unable to predict the overall outcome. We can, however, surmise a number of possible phases patients may experience. Figure 19.1 outlines these different phases which can help healthcare professionals to identify support and services that patients might need at different points.

Depending on the type of cancer/palliative care placement (hub or spoke) you have been allocated to, you may care for patients at a specific stage in the cancer experience. For instance, if you are on an oncology ward, you may experience patients receiving cancer treatments and undergoing a review of their symptom management.

It is worthwhile to read all of the chapters in the case study. This gives you an insight into what patients have experienced prior to their current situation, as well as what might be ahead of them. It is also a good idea to arrange some insight visits to some of

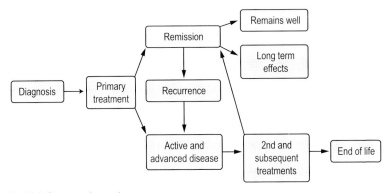

Fig 19.1 Cancer patient pathway

the other clinical environments within the pathway. To help you do this, go back to Section 2 to identify other cancer/palliative care treatments and experiences.

Case study introduction

Michelle is a 44-year-old woman who has been diagnosed with a non-specific type of breast cancer. She is married to Simon with three children, aged 8, 11 and 16. Michelle works part time as a receptionist at a GP surgery. Her parents and parents-in-law live a considerable distance away and are in their mid-70s. Michelle has a good network of friends locally and she attends a gym. She is a Catholic but her beliefs and religious practices in that faith have not been adhered to and she admits she is a 'lapsed Catholic'.

The remaining chapters focus on the following:
- Chapter 20: Michelle receives her diagnosis and discusses treatment options.
- Chapter 21: she experiences treatment and associated complications.
- Chapter 22: she develops complex symptoms associated with advancing disease.
- Chapters 23 and 24: two alternative endings to Michelle's cancer experience.
- Chapter 23: as Michelle's disease advances, we explore palliation of her symptoms and care as she moves towards receiving last days of life care.
- Chapter 24: the final pathway explores how she makes the transition to living beyond cancer.

20 Receiving a cancer diagnosis

Michelle finds a lump in her left breast while she is in the shower. It doesn't hurt when she touches it, so she thinks it might result from hormone changes during her monthly menstrual cycle and decides to wait a few weeks to see if it disappears. A couple of weeks later the lump hasn't gone so she makes an appointment with her GP. Her GP examines her and tells her that he is unsure of what the lump is, that it might be a simple cyst, but he would like to refer her to a specialist for further tests.

Michelle attends an appointment with a breast specialist, accompanied by Simon.

The consultant reassures her that although he doesn't know what the lump is at this stage, he will need to conduct a 'triple assessment', involving clinical, radiological and pathological evaluation of both her breasts. First, a clinical examination is performed and a clinical history is taken. Michelle then has a mammogram and an ultrasound of both breasts. She has an ultrasound-guided core biopsy of the lump, under a local anaesthetic, to obtain tissue for pathology. Michelle also has a blood test to check for the presence of tumour markers.

 Activity

Diagnostic investigations

Make a list of what the consultant may want to know about Michelle's personal and family history. Consider how this information might influence the management of her cancer.

Recall an experience of observing a patient having a specific investigation (a scan, X-ray, biopsy, etc.). Write a short reflective piece on how the patient was prepared (physically and mentally); how safety and patient comfort was maintained; what the advantages of this investigation were; what the potential risks were; and how the specimen (if taken) was processed.

Think about what Michelle's concerns might be while she is undergoing the tests and while she is waiting for the results. How can a healthcare professional support Michelle during these procedures? What specific information might Michelle need once the results from the triple assessment have been gathered?

Register with the free Macmillan 'Learn Zone' on the following Website: http://learnzone.macmillan.org.uk (accessed November 2011).

Follow the tab to the 'health and social care professionals' section and scroll down to the 'information giving' course and work through the exercises.

NMC Domain 1: 1.6
NMC Domain 2: 2.1; 2.2; 2.3; 2.4; 2.7
NMC Domain 3: 3.1; 3.3; 3.4; 3.8

Further reading

Johnson, G.B., 2007. Cancer diagnosis and staging. In: Langhorne, M.E., Fulton, J.S., Otto, S.E. (Eds.), Oncology nursing. fifth ed. Mosby, St Louis.

Montgomery, M., McCrone, S., 2010. Psychological distress associated with the diagnostic phase for suspected breast cancer: systematic review. J. Adv. Nurs. 66 (11), 2372–2390.

Points to consider

A medical history attempts to identify relevant information that might provide clues to what the lump may be. It may also highlight any risk factors such as inherited cancer patterns or lifestyles behaviours, as well as many other factors that might influence treatment options.

Without pathology, a diagnosis cannot be made. Further diagnostic investigations are essential to identify the type, exact location, grade and stage to ensure appropriate treatment is delivered. Although the time period between seeing the consultant and receiving the results is only a matter of days, 2 weeks at the most, for the majority of patients it is a very scary time. It is often the 'not knowing' that is particularly difficult to deal with and a number of patients feel a sense of relief once a diagnosis has been confirmed (even if it is a cancer diagnosis).

Case update

Once all the investigations have been completed, Michelle returns to the clinic accompanied by Simon to hear the results. The consultant and breast nurse specialist check Michelle and Simon's understanding about why the investigations were done and what they thought might be causing the lump. Michelle is told she has a 'non-special type' (NST) of breast cancer. Hearing this news, Michelle feels stunned and is in a state of shock: 'How could she have cancer? She felt so well!'

The consultant gives them some time on their own, to digest the information. The nurse specialist then spends some time with them to reiterate and explain what had been said and answer any questions they have. When they feel able, Michelle and Simon return to the consultant to discuss the treatment options. The consultant suggests that Michelle has either a wide local excision (segment of breast removed) or a simple mastectomy (removal of the entire breast) with the option of an optional breast reconstruction immediately or later, and 5 weeks of radiotherapy. He discusses the advantages and disadvantages of both. Michelle decides to have a simple mastectomy, but wants to think about breast reconstruction at a later date.

Activity

Receiving a diagnosis and decision making

Write a reflection of an observation where significant news was delivered. This may be a diagnosis, prognosis or disease progression. Reflect on the individual's reactions to the news and the strategies that the healthcare professional used to give the information.

Refer back to Chapter 8. What would the consultant and Michelle have considered when deciding on treatment options?

NMC Domain 1: 1.2; 1.4; 1.5; 1.6; 1.9
NMC Domain 2: 2.1; 2.2; 2.3; 2.4; 2.5
NMC Domain 3: 3.6; 3.9; 3.10

Further reading

Fujimorl, M., Uchitomi, Y., 2009. Preferences of cancer patients regarding communication of bad news: a systematic literature review. J. Clin. Oncol. 39 (4), 201–216.

Thain, C., Palmer, C., 2010. Strategies to ensure effective and empathetic delivery of bad news. Cancer Nursing Practice 9 (9), 24–27.

Points to consider

For most individuals, hearing the news they have cancer is a shock, even if they suspected the diagnosis or if healthcare professionals had previously suggested this might be the cause of their symptoms. Often patients do not hear any information that is given straight after the diagnosis which is why it is important to give them time for the news to sink in before discussing treatment options. Not all patients will want to be solely responsible for treatment decision making and it is important that healthcare professionals discusse with the patient how much they would like to be involved in the decision. It is worth noting that patients may wish to take a greater role in decision making as time progresses, depending on the nature of the decision, and healthcare professionals need to constantly gauge patient involvement desire.

 Activity

Preoperative care

When consenting Michelle for her surgical procedure, what is the healthcare professional considering? Write a short outline of the main legal, ethical and professional aspects of accountability during the consent process. What information will Michelle need to sign the consent form?

When completing Michelle's preoperative assessment, what do you consider the priorities of her care to be? Compare this to another patient who has undergone surgery. How similar are these and what influences the preoperative care required?

NMC Domain 1: 1.1; 1.2; 1.4; 1.7
NMC Domain 2: 2.1; 2.2 2.3; 2.7; 2.8
NMC Domain 3: 3.1; 3.3; 3.4; 3.6;
3.8; 3.10
NMC Domain 4: 4.3

Further reading

Caulfield, H., 2005. Vital notes for nurses: accountability. Wiley-Blackwell, Edinburgh.

Ford, L., 2010. Consent and capacity: a guide for district nurses. Br. J. Community Nurs. 15 (9), 456–460.

Mental Capacity Act. 2005. The Stationery Office, London.

Pudner, R., 2010. Nursing the surgical patient, third ed. Baillière Tindall, Edinburgh.

Points to consider

The preoperative period can be full of mixed emotions. Patients often feel anxious about having a general anaesthetic and can be distressed anticipating the loss of a breast. A number of patients feel relieved that, after the wait for the results, progress is being made and the cancer will be removed.

The majority will be concerned with the final pathology and the lymph node biopsy report.

Preoperative assessment is essential to identify any existing physical or psychological factors that may hamper the surgical procedure or the patient's recovery. It is also important that the patient is prepared for theatre correctly to ensure patient safety.

21 Receiving treatment

Case update

Two weeks after diagnosis, Michelle undergoes a left mastectomy. During the surgery, a sentinel node biopsy is taken to see if the cancer has spread to any of Michelle's axillary lymph nodes. Two of the nodes are found to be positive. Immediately after surgery, the tissue that was removed from Michelle's breast is tested for receptors, to see if the cancer is responsive to hormones (oestrogen and/or progesterone) and to see if there is overexpression of HER2 receptors. She is found to have an oestrogen-positive cancer, however the cancer is *not* overexpressing HER2 receptors nor is it progesterone responsive. The cancer is then staged as follows:

- The size of the cancer was 2 cm in diameter.
- Two lymph nodes (glands) were positive under the arm.

- The grade of the cancer (how aggressive the cancer is) was assessed to be grade II (intermediate aggressive in appearance).

The Nottingham Prognostic Index (NPI) is calculated as 4.4. This means that Michelle has an intermediate chance of being cured. She will, therefore, require adjuvant treatment to reduce the risk of recurrence.

Michelle makes a swift recovery from the operation and is able to go home the following day to recuperate. Before her discharge, she is seen by the breast nurse specialist who fits Michelle with a soft prosthesis which slips into her bra. She can wear this as soon as she feels comfortable. The breast nurse arranges an appointment for Michelle to return for a proper prosthetic fitting as an outpatient. She is also seen by the physiotherapist who teaches her some arm exercises that she should do daily to maintain the strength and flexibility in her left shoulder and arm.

 Activity

Postoperative care

Summarise the main physiological processes involved in wound healing. Identify the most conducive environment to prompt healing following a surgical procedure.

Write a care plan for Michelle's immediate postoperative care required.

Consider the importance of accurate and thorough documentation of healthcare activity and events. Refer to the Nursing and Midwifery Council (2009) *Record Keeping: Guidance for Nurses and Midwives*:

http://www.nmc-uk.org/Documents/Guidance/nmcGuidanceRecordKeeping GuidanceforNursesandMidwives.pdf (accessed November 2011)

NMC Domain 1: 1.2; 1.3; 1.4; 1.5; 1.6; 1.9
NMC Domain 3: 3.1; 3.2; 3.3; 3.4; 3.5; 3.6; 3.7; 3.8; 3.9; 3.10

Further reading

Hughes, E., 2004. Principles of post-operative patient care. Nurs. Stand 19 (5), 43–51, 53, 56.

Thompson, A.M., Wells, M., 2006. Surgery. In: Kearney, N., Richardson, A. (Eds.), Nursing patients with cancer: principles and practice. Churchill Livingstone, Edinburgh.

Points to consider

The postoperative period can be extremely challenging. There are many immediate and long-term issues to deal with. Directly after surgery, the focus must be on the physical health status of the patient: oxygenation of tissues; respiratory and cardiovascular function; fluid balance; infection control; pain management; body temperature, etc. These all need careful monitoring. There are many implications of surgery in the longer terms, such as adapting to the physical appearance and/or the physical function. These may be unexpected (even if the patient was informed preoperatively) and can be extremely difficult to deal with.

 Activity

Discharge

Draft a discharge plan for Michelle, or identify a patient who you have discharged home following a hospital admission, and reflect on the planning involved. Consider: what rehabilitation do they require? Are there any household alterations required before discharge? Which other multiprofessionals need to be involved? What information does the patient and their family need? Is transport required? What medications does the patient need once at home? Are any referrals to community services required?

NMC Domain 1: 1.2; 1.3; 1.4; 1.6
NMC Domain 2:2.1; 2.2; 2.3; 2.4; 2.6; 2.7; 2.8
NMC Domain 3: 3.1; 3.3; 3.4 3.5; 3.8; 3.9; 3.10
NMC Domain 4: 4.7

Further reading

Royal College of Nursing, 2004. Day surgery: discharge information. Online. Available at: http://www.rcn.org.uk/__data/assets/pdf_file/0011/78509/001376.pdf (accessed May 2011).

Points to consider

The transition from hospital to home can be quite anxious for most patients. Leaving the security of the specialised healthcare environment can feel isolating and scary. Patients need good information about: who to call if they experience any complications; what they should/should not do once they get home; what rehabilitation exercises will assist their recovery; which medications they should take and how often; when they need any sutures/clips removed and who will do this; when they need to return for a follow-up appointment, etc. Although most patients prefer tailored information, there is so much information to take in that patients should be given a written record as well.

The role of the nurse is essential in providing supportive care. As hospital stays decrease, there is an increased need for community nurses to become more knowledgeable and skilled in caring for postoperative patients.

 Activity

Psychological impact of surgery

Think about the changes in Michelle's body appearance after the loss of a breast. How might her perception of her body alter? How might this affect her confidence and sexuality as well as her social situation?

Write a reflection on an observation/experience you have encountered where a patient underwent surgery and their body image was altered. What could have been done to minimise this impact and what can be done to aid adjustment?

Register on Macmillan's 'Learn Zone' on their Website:

http://learnzone.macmillan.org.uk (accessed November 2011)

Follow the tabs to the 'Health and social care professionals' section, scroll down to the 'Body image' course and work through the exercises.

Think about what might be concerning Simon regarding his relationship with Michelle. Find an article that considers how partners might feel when their spouse has undergone surgery.

NMC Domain 1: 1.2; 1.3; 1.5; 1.6; 1.9
NMC Domain 2: 2.1; 2.2; 2.3; 2.4; 2.6
NMC Domain 3: 3.1; 3.3; 3.4; 3.5; 3.8; 3.9; 3.10
NMC Domain 4: 4.2

Further reading

Chan, L., 2010. Body image and the breast: the psychological wound. J. Wound Care 19 (4), 133–138.

Price, B., 2009. Understanding patient accounts of body image change. Cancer Nursing Practice 8 (6), 29–34.

Points to consider

The time patients spend in hospital postoperatively is very brief, therefore it is important to prioritise their needs while they are on the ward and plan discharge from the outset. Depending on patients' needs and the surgical procedure they have undergone, close liaison with other agencies, such as the GP, community nurses, occupational therapies, physiotherapists, pharmacists, social workers, etc., is paramount to ensure patients are safely discharged and supported once at home.

Partners, family members and informal carers can find it particularly difficult and confusing once the patient is discharged home. It is a daunting prospect being a carer: not knowing what to expect, worrying that the patient may be in pain and that you are being depended upon. There is often a temptation to want to smother or wrap the patient in cotton wool. This can be frustrating for the patient who may want to regain independence as soon as they are physically able, and may feel that their rehabilitation is hampered. It can also be difficult for partners to feel physically close to the patient, even when wounds have healed. They may fear causing pain or harm to the patient. Sometimes these anxieties continue for a significant length of time and can affect relationships and feelings of intimacy in the long term.

Further reading

Foubert, J., Vaessen, G., 2005. Nausea: the neglected symptom? Eur. J. Oncol. Nurs. 9, 21–32.

Molassiotis, A., Stricker, C.T., Easby, B., et al., 2008. Understanding the concept of chemotherapy related nausea: the patient experience. Eur. J. Cancer 17, 444–453.

 Activity

Cytotoxic therapy

Look up and make a list of the side effects of 5-FU, epirubicin and cyclophosphamide. What side effects is Michelle likely to experience? Identify strategies that prevent/minimise these toxicities.

Write a reflection on one or two patients you have cared for while, or after, they received cytotoxic therapy. What toxicities did they encounter? How were these assessed and managed?

What antiemetic is Michelle likely to be prescribed alongside this regimen?

What advice should Michelle be given to reduce her chances of getting an infection while she is receiving cytotoxic treatment?

What signs and symptoms of infection should Michelle look out for? Who do patients need to inform in your area if they suspect they have a temperature?

How might Michelle feel about losing her hair? What are the local arrangements for patients to obtain a wig? Find out about scalp cooling in your area.

What might the financial and social implications be of Michelle having to take time away from work?

NMC Domain 1: 1.2; 1.3; 1.4; 1.5; 1.6; 1.7; 1.8; 1.9
NMC Domain 2: 2.1; 2.2; 2.3; 2.4; 2.5; 2.6
NMC Domain 3: 3.1; 3.2; 3.3; 3.4; 3.6; 3.7; 3.8; 3.9; 3.10
NMC Domain 4: 4.1; 4.2; 4.3

Case update

Michelle recovers well from her surgery and returns for her postoperative follow-up appointment. The results from the sentinel node biopsy and endocrine response are explained and Michelle is referred to the oncologist to receive six courses of chemotherapy – 5- fluorouracil (5-FU), epirubicin and cyclophosphamide (FEC). Given every 3 weeks, this will take approximately 5 months. She is given a date to meet with the chemotherapy nurse practitioner to discuss the possible side effects of the drugs and what she needs to know to stay well through her treatment. The nurse highlights that, during treatment, Michelle's immune system will be reduced making her prone to infection. Therefore, Michelle is advised not to go to the GP practice where she works as it is a likely source of infection. Michelle returns to see the oncologist to sign a consent form and have a number of blood tests taken. A date is set for her to commence treatment.

Michelle attends the outpatient clinic the day before each cycle to see the chemotherapy nurse practitioner to check she is coping with the treatment and to have her pretreatment blood tests taken. On the day of treatment, a peripheral cannula is sited and antiemetic drugs and cytotoxic drugs are infused over 45 minutes.

Points to consider

There is a lot of information for patients to take in at the beginning of cytotoxic treatment. It is important that contact telephone numbers are given and written information is provided to refer to once at home. Information is needed so the patient and carer know what to expect and how to manage any toxicities that may occur. In particular, how to reduce infection risk is essential: meticulous hand washing; thorough aseptic care of the central venous access device (CVAD); good personal and dental hygiene; avoiding contact with other individuals with coughs/colds and crowded places; maintaining nutrition; avoiding rectal examination and medication; avoiding clearing up pet faeces; and avoiding taking antipyrexial drugs such as paracetamol. They will also need guidance on their antiemetic medication.

Patients often think that the toxicities from cytotoxic treatment are inevitable and that they have to endure them. There is also a real fear for patients that if they do report problems then the treatment will be stopped. For instance, cytotoxic-induced nausea and vomiting is intrinsically associated with chemotherapy, therefore patients expect to feel sick and do not report nausea and vomiting, but a simple adjustment of antiemetics may resolve the situation.

Reporting any adverse side effects of treatment is vital so intervention can be prompt. Patients must know who to contact and they need to do this as a matter of urgency.

Having adjuvant treatment can be difficult as patients often feel they have recovered from surgery and are beginning to re-establish a routine. It can be very time-consuming with numerous visits to the hospital.

Case update

Ten days after the second cycle of treatment, Michelle's mouth starts to feel sore and she notices a few ulcers at the bottom of her mouth. She also doesn't feel very well generally. She checks her temperature and discovers that she has a temperature of 38.2°C. She contacts the chemotherapy unit and is admitted to the oncology ward for intravenous (IV) antibiotics.

 Activity

Neutropenic sepsis

Make a list of the factors that may contribute to making Michelle and other cancer patients so susceptible to infection.

When admitting a patient with suspected neutropenic sepsis, how and what would you assess? What would the signs and symptoms of sepsis be?

Find out what the neutropenic policy and protocol is in your area.

NMC Domain 1: 1.3
NMC Domain 3: 3.1; 3.2; 3.3; 3.4; 3.6; 3.7; 3.8; 3.9; 3.10
NMC Domain 4: 4.2; 4.3

Further reading

Brighton, D., Wood, M., 2005. The Royal Marsden Hospital handbook of cancer chemotherapy. Churchill Livingstone, Edinburgh.

Coughlan, M., Healy, C., 2008. Nursing care, education and support for patients with neutropenia. Nurs. Stand. 22 (46), 35–41.

Points to consider

Neutropenia is a potentially life-threatening side effect of cytotoxic therapy. It is vitally important that patients report signs and symptoms of infection and receive IV antibiotics *within 1 hour* of arriving at hospital; this is known as the 'door to needle

time'. Because the mortality rates from neutropenic sepsis are very high in cancer patients, you need to act quickly when you are admitting the patient with suspected neutropenic sepsis. A thorough assessment is needed:

- Observations: temperature, blood pressure, pulse, respirations, oxygen saturations, peripheral refill.
- Look at the patient's skin colour, as well as the site of infection: wounds, CVAD sites, breaks in the skin or mucosa. The classic signs of infection – redness, warmth, pain, raised temperature – may or may not be present. Pus may not be present. This is because, if there is a lack of neutrophills, there will not be enough phagocytes to engulf the pathogen and produce the byproduct which is pus.
- Get a good history of the last few days: when cytotoxic treatment was last received; evidence of frequency or discomfort passing urine; persistent cough or cold; diarrhoea; pain, etc.
- Take blood for cultures (peripheral and from a CVAD if in place), full blood count and biochemistry, as well as specimens and swabs of any area of the body that may be the likely site of infection (urinalysis; mid-stream urine specimen; swab CVAD sites; sputum specimen if cough present; stool specimen if diarrhoea; throat swab if sore).

In many cancer centres, intravenous broad-spectrum antibiotics for neutropenic patients are covered by patient group directions (PGD) and are given directly after blood cultures are taken. If the patient is hypotensive then intravenous fluids will be required. Careful fluid balance measurement is needed to monitor renal function and ensure hydration. The patient will need frequent observations, depending on their status and condition. Many hospitals use an early warning score (EWS) to trigger critical care interventions if the patient starts to deteriorate.

Even with IV support and antibiotics, it may take some time for a patient's condition to improve. This is dependent on the degree and duration of neutropenia; type and number of pathogens; the site of entry; the presence of co-morbidity; and the promptness of intervention. In addition, patients may not respond to the prescribed antibiotics, which may indicate resistant pathogens, multiple pathogens (such as viral or fungal agents) or insufficient serum levels of antibiotics (especially gentamycin and vancomycin). A regular medical review of the patient's progress should be made, to alter or adjust treatment as needed.

If the patient's neutrophil count has not reached 2×10^9/L by the time they are due the next cycle of chemotherapy, this may delay cytotoxic treatment significantly. If this happens on a number of occassions, then colony-stimulating factors such as filgrastim (G-CSF) might be used to boost the white blood cells to ensure subsequent cycles are delivered on schedule.

 Activity

Mucositis

Think about an experience while on placement where you have performed or observed an oral assessment. What was assessed and how was the patient's mouth assessed?

Find out whether your local practice area uses an oral assessment tool. If so, find out how to use this and how this links to the management of mucositis. What is the evidence base behind the oral protocol?

NMC Domain 1: 1.4; 1.9
NMC Domain 3: 3.1; 3.2; 3.3; 3.4; 3.7; 3.8; 3.10
NMC Domain 4: 4.2

Further reading

Maxwell, C.J., 2008. Putting evidence into practice: evidence-based interventions for the management of oral mucositis. Clin. J. Oncol. Nurs. 12 (1), 141–152.

McGowan, D., 2008. Chemotherapy-induced oral dysfunction: a literature review. Br. J. Nurs. 17 (22), 1422–1426.

Points to consider

Oral mucositis can affect the patient in many ways, physically (route of infection, reduced nutritional and fluid intake, compromised communication, pain) as well as psychosocially (reduced physical closeness with loved ones, change in body image, etc.) Pretreatment assessment is important to establish a benchmark to compare potential changes with. Assessment tools provide nurses with a guide, prompting them to conduct a systematic assessment, however the assessment tool must then be used to identify specific intervention to improve the oral cavity. Regular reassessment is required to monitor severity and impact of mucositis.

Case update

Michelle spends 4 days in hospital having intravenous antibiotics and fluids. Her temperature returns to normal and her neutrophil count increases slowly. She is discharged home and completes the remaining four cycles of cytotoxic therapy without problems.

Three weeks after completing cytotoxic therapy, Michelle commences a 5-week course of radiotherapy. She has a computed tomography CT scan to plan her treatment and spends time with one of the radiographers, who explains how the treatment works and what she should expect while having treatment. She attends the radiotherapy department daily (Monday to Friday).

 Activity

Radiotherapy

Reflect on an insight visit to the radiotherapy department. What were your first impressions of the environment and the machinery? How might this make the patient feel on their first visit?

Recall what the main side effects of radiotherapy are. What specific problems might Michelle experience while she is having radiotherapy to her breast? What care should Michelle take to minimise the side effects? How might the daily appointments affect Michelle's family and social life?

NMC Domain 1: 1.2; 1.3; 1.4; 1.5; 1.5; 1.6; 1.7
NMC Domain 3: 3.1; 3.2; 3.6; 3.7; 3.8

Points to consider

Although enhanced radiotherapy planning techniques have improved the accuracy of treatment and reduced the incidence, severity and duration of side effects, patients still commonly experience radiation skin reactions.

The acute side effects of radiotherapy may take a number of weeks before they present, and may last long after treatment has concluded. So it is important that patients are informed of the likely time span of adverse side effects, who to report them to and how to minimise the severity of the reaction. Gently washing and drying the area is essential; wearing natural fibres; avoiding sun light; and moisturising help minimise the severity of the reaction.

Activity

Radiotherapy toxicities

Refresh your knowledge by recalling the normal skin renewal timing and process. How is this disrupted in radiotherapy?

Write a reflection on an experience caring for a patient undergoing or having finished radiotherapy. What toxicities did they encounter and how did this affect them psychosocially, physically and economically? What supportive care was offered?

Find out what the local radiotherapy skin care protocols are in your area.

Find out what strategies help with cancer-related and cancer treatment-related fatigue.

What might the impact on the family be if Michelle is unable to continue her role as mother and wife?

Why might Michelle feel anxious coming to the end of treatment?

NMC Domain 1: 1.2; 1.3; 1.4; 1.5
NMC Domain 2: 2.1; 2.2; 2.3; 2.4; 2.6
NMC Domain 3: 3.1; 3.2; 3.3; 3.4; 3.5; 3.7; 3.8; 3.10
NMC Domain 4: 4.2

Further reading

Sjovall, K., Strombeck, G., Lofgren, A., 2010. Adjuvant radiotherapy of women with breast cancer: information, support and side-effects. Eur. J. Oncol. Nurs. 14 (2), 147–153.

Case update

Two weeks after starting radiotherapy, Michelle's skin within the radiotherapy field starts to feel taut and tender to touch and slightly red.

For the first few weeks, Michelle drives to the hospital herself, but after 3 weeks she is feeling extremely tired and is finding it very difficult to cope with family life and the travelling to and from the hospital. In particular, she finds the daily school run exhausting and is falling asleep during the day. During her last week of radiotherapy, Michelle starts to feel anxious and emotional.

Points to consider

Radiation skin reactions can be severe. A number of patients experience moist desquamation (where the skin integrity is lost significantly) and have their treatment postponed for a few days; this may reduce the efficacy of treatment.

Radiotherapy can be an arduous emotional and physical experience. The daily visits can be exhausting and can affect an individual's ability to drive back and forth to the radiotherapy department as well as other day-to-day activities. Radiotherapy-related fatigue is difficult to manage as little can be done to reduce the unrelenting feeling of exhaustion. Ironically, exercise can help – doing 30 minutes of gentle/moderate exercise (like walking) can reduce the severity of tiredness. Planning and spacing out daily activities can help, scheduling a rest between small tasks. Accepting additional help with domestic tasks can be frustrating and psychologically challenging, with the loss of an individual's independence, but can often be necessary to help preserve social role by preserving energy. For instance, having help with cleaning the house may allow an individual to focus energy on cooking a family meal.

Case update

Once Michelle has completed her radiotherapy, she returns to the oncologist for a post-treatment follow up. The oncologist is pleased with her progress and, although there are no signs of disease, he commences her on tamoxifen 20 mg daily for 5 years, as her cancer was oestrogen responsive. She is now considered disease free. Michelle will now be seen in the follow-up clinic every year for 5 years and will have an annual mammogram until she is 50 years old.

Points to consider

As endocrine therapy is taken orally and patients usually self-manage at home, the side effects of treatment are often under-reported and underestimated by healthcare professionals. Patients can experience severe toxicities which last for many years and they often don't know who they should tell. Because many of the side effects affect the normal gender hormones, the patient may experience changes in their appearance and sexual functioning. For instance, it is common for male patients to experience impotence, loss of sexual desire and increased breast growth. Females may experience loss of libido, vaginal dryness and hot flushes. Patients often find these effects difficult to discuss with healthcare professionals, so it is important that healthcare professionals provide an appropriately private environment and sensitively raise the issue of such side effects, giving the patient permission to talk about any problems they may be encountering. Some patients may not wish to discuss such matters and will change the conversation, which should be respected.

Activity

Endocrine therapy

Look up the toxicities of tamoxifen. Reflect on patients you may have cared for who were prescribed endocrine treatment. What side effects did they experience? What strategies can be used to help manage these adverse effects?

NMC Domain 3: 3.1; 3.2; 3.3; 3.4; 3.5; 3.7; 3.8; 3.10

Points to consider

Having completed treatment, patients are discharged home to adjust and adapt to their change of health status, which may have resulted from the cancer and/or treatment. This can be a particularly anxious time for patients, especially after the flurry of tests and treatments and the many appointments at the hospital. Patients may sit at home, not knowing what to do with themselves. They may experience major physical effects such as loss of mobility; breathlessness; fatigue; reduced nutritional intake; and gastrointestinal functioning may be disrupted as well as many more. This might mean they are not fit enough to return to previous employment and hobbies. Their social contacts may also be diminished. Many patients express feeling lost or 'in limbo' at this stage and it may take some time for them to adjust. They will still attend regular outpatient appointments to be monitored, however follow-up visits rarely help reduce patient anxieties (often adding to them). Telephone follow up is becoming increasingly popular. This is where a nurse specialist makes a pre-arranged phone call to the patient to enquire about their progress and to see if they require any additional support.

The next three chapters explore two very different possible paths Michelle's story may take. Chapters 22 and 23 explore the situation where Michelle presents with secondary disease and her prognosis is poor. Chapter 23 offers an alternative ending, in which Michelle remains disease free and lives a healthy life beyond cancer. Statistically, this is the most likely outcome, reflecting the 82% of all women diagnosed with breast cancer who survive 5 years and 73% of women who survive 10 years (Rachet et al 2009).

 Activity

Follow up

Consider who will be primarily responsible for Michelle's health care. Who should she seek help from if she requires advice or help?

Find out how the cancer specialist team in the acute care setting (oncologist and nurse specialists) communicate with the primary health team in the community (GP and practice nurse).

NMC Domain 1: 1.5; 1.6
NMC Domain 4: 4.6; 4.10

Reference

Rachet, B., Maringe, C., Nur, U., et al., 2009. Population-based cancer survival trends in England and Wales up to 2007: an assessment of the NHS cancer plan for England. Lancet Oncology 10 (4), 351–369.

Further reading

Cooley, C., 2010. Cancer survivorship, part 1: how services need to change for those living with and beyond cancer. Nurs. Times 106 (20), 24–25.

Cox, K., Wilson, E., 2003. Follow-up for people with cancer: nurse led services and telephone interventions. J. Adv. Nurs. 43 (1), 51–61.

Office for National Statistics, 2007. Survival rates in England, patients diagnosed 2001–2006. ONS, London.

Pennery, E., 2008. The role of endocrine therapies in reducing risk of recurrence in postmenopausal women with hormone receptor-positive breast cancer. Eur. J. Oncol. Nurs. 12 (3), 233–243.

22 Advancing disease

Case update

It is 8 months since Michelle received her last treatment and was discharged from the oncology ward. After resting for 2 months, Michelle returned to her role as a doctors' receptionist for 5 hours per week. Returning to work is important to Michelle, especially being able to get dressed and put on her make-up. Her hair has grown back and Michelle has had it restyled – her family and friends think it looks 'fab'. Michelle has felt continuously tired and has put this down to returning to work and 'dealing with the diagnosis'. She has visited her GP several times who has monitored her recovery.

Michelle has been feeling increasingly unwell over the last 4 weeks and is getting quite distressed at home. This is mainly due to nausea and vomiting, tiredness and not feeling rested after sleep, with increasing abdominal pain, back pain and reduced mobility. Michelle has been in bed for 6 days and feels too unwell for Simon to take her in the car to visit her GP, so he does a home visit. She feels too tired to help with the children's homework and is very tearful.

Her GP recognises the deterioration in Michelle's condition and arranges for her to be admitted to the local medical admission unit for urgent assessment and management of her symptoms. He starts her on morphine 10 mg as required to help her feel more comfortable while waiting for the admission. Michelle appears relieved at this decision to be admitted and is taken to hospital by ambulance on that same day. The only other medication Michelle has been taking is a hormone relating to her breast cancer treatment.

Simon is very tired and feeling frustrated that he doesn't seem to be able to help her distress. The children are getting to school late and Simon has not been to work for the last week.

 Activity

Assessment and holistic care

Complete the family assessment tool introduced in Appendix 2. This will assist you to gather information about Simon and the other family members so you can start to make an assessment as to how they are coping with the changing situation.

Make a list of what you think the main concerns and worries might be for:

- Simon
- the children
- Michelle's parents.

What do you think their current understanding of Michelle's illness is?

As the nurse looking after Michelle, consider what your main concerns would be.

Make a list of the other information that is needed to make a holistic assessment of Michelle.

NMC Domain 1: 1.1; 1.2; 1.4
NMC Domain 2: 2.1; 2.3; 2.4
NMC Domain 3: 3.1; 3.3; 3.7; 3.9
NMC Domain 4: 4.3

Further reading

Maher, D., Hemming, L., 2005. Understanding patient and family: holistic assessment and palliative care. Br. J. Community Nurs. 10 (7), 318–322.

Taylor, E., 2007. Supporting families of dying patients: communication skills. End of Life Care 1 (3), 8–15.

Points to consider

Information collected on admission can be useful when planning a complex discharge, and completing the admission assessment documentation as fully as possible provides a lot of core information. For example, Michelle had reduced mobility before the admission so it is important to find out where the bathroom is at home. If access to a toilet has been a problem before admission, it is essential this is given consideration for the discharge planning process. It is also important to find out what medications have been prescribed and not to assume they have been taken by Michelle. Ensure all this information is clearly documented so any person from the care team helping to arrange discharge has the correct information.

Case update

A magnetic resonance imaging (MRI) scan and blood tests have shown that Michelle's disease has progressed and the abdominal pain is from spinal metastases. Her blood calcium is raised, giving the diagnosis of hypercalcaemia. Michelle and Simon are now given this difficult news.

 Activity

Breaking bad/significant news

This is significantly bad news for both Michelle and Simon and consideration is needed of how this news will be given. Access the East Midlands Cancer Network 'Guidelines for communicating bad news':

http://www.eastmidlandscancernet work.nhs.uk/Library/Breaking BadNewsGuidelines.pdf (accessed November 2011).

You will find an 11-step flowchart on page 32. For each of the 11 steps, write down how you can prepare to give this significant news to Michelle and Simon. Who might be the best person to give this news? If you were giving the news, consider how you would prepare.

NMC Domain 1: 1.1; 1.2
NMC Domain 2: 2.1; 2.2; 2.4; 2.5
NMC Domain 3: 3.7; 3.8
NMC Domain 4.4; 4.6

Further reading

Fujimorl, M., Uchitomi, Y., 2009. Preferences of cancer patients regarding communication of bad news: a systematic literature review. J. Clin. Oncol. 39 (4), 201–216.

Girgis, A., Sanson-Fisher, R., Schofield, M., 1999. Is there consensus between breast cancer patients and providers on guidelines for breaking bad news? Behav. Med 25 (2), 69–77.

Points to consider

Receiving news about a change in condition can be as devastating as receiving news at the time of the original cancer diagnosis. Where possible, ensure that all members of the care team are aware the news is being given so they can offer support, not only to the patient and their family but also to those in the care team who are giving the information.

We now consider what might be causing each of the symptoms Michelle is experiencing.

 Activity

Back pain

Advancing disease is the most likely reason for Michelle's back pain. Refer to Section 2 and read again about malignant spinal cord compression.

Is it expected for a breast cancer diagnosis? Is there anything unusual in Michelle having spinal cord compression now? What are the first two things the nursing team will need to do to ensure Michelle's comfort?

Now write a plan for Michelle to help manage her spinal cord compression.

NMC Domain 1: 1.1; 1.2
NMC Domain 2: 2.2; 2.4
NMC Domain 3: 3.1; 3.2; 3.7; 3.9
NMC Domain 4: 4.1

Further reading

Drudge-Coates, L., Rajbabul, K., 2008. Diagnosis and management of malignant cord compression: part 1. Int. J. Palliat. Nurs. 14 (3), 110–116.

Drudge-Coates, L., Rajbabul, K., 2008. Diagnosis and management of malignant cord compression: part 2. Int. J. Palliat. Nurs. 14 (4), 175–180.

Morgan, H., Cawley, D., 2009. Recognising metastatic spinal cord compression and treatment. End of Life Care 3 (4), 15–21.

Points to consider

Malignant spinal cord compression is a significant and distressing symptom since it can drastically impact on a patient's activities of living as well as signify a serious advance of the cancer. Patients and their families need much support and care at this time.

 Activity

Nausea and vomiting

Refer back to the seven vomiting pathways in Section 2. For each vomiting pathway, jot down the information your care team will need to gather to make a correct assessment of Michelle's changing condition.

Consider what information you already have about Michelle which can be used in your assessment.

It is likely that the nausea is being caused by hypercalcaemia and anxiety, so the vomiting pathways involved are:

- chemically-induced nausea (from the calcium and morphine) stimulating the chemoreceptor trigger zone
- anxiety stimulating the cerebral cortex.

Refer back to page 139 on managing symptoms to refresh your knowledge on how this symptom is managed.

Make a note of the drug(s) Michelle might now be prescribed. If these drugs are new to you, look up how they work. This will help you to link the care to the physiology of vomiting. Also look up any side effects of these drugs so care can be planned appropriately.

NMC Domain 1: 1.1; 1.2
NMC Domain 2: 2.2; 2.4
NMC Domain 3: 3.2; 3.7; 3.9
NMC Domain 4: 4.1

Further reading

Campbell, T., Hately, J., 2000. The management of nausea and vomiting in advanced cancer. Int. J. Palliat. Nurs. 6 (1), 18–25.

Points to consider

A patient who is not vomiting can be very distressed from unresolved nausea. It is important to ask how the patient is feeling and not to make the assumption that no vomiting means no nausea.

 Activity

Abdominal pain

This can be related to both the hypercalcaemia, due to increased plasma calcium, and the administration of morphine. Re-read about constipation on page 144 to refresh your memory of causes and management.

What is the link between morphine and abdominal pain? Why is it important to know the medication that Michelle has been prescribed and to establish if she has taken it? Why do we need to know about Michelle's (a) normal bowel habit and (b) recent bowel habit? What medication does Michelle need to be started on?

Now write down two or three sentences you might use if you were explaining to Michelle and Simon about her abdominal pain and why it is important to take laxatives while on morphine.

NMC Domain 1: 1.1; 1.2
NMC Domain 2: 2.2; 2.4
NMC Domain 3: 3.2; 3.7; 3.9
NMC Domain 4: 4.1

Further reading

Kyle, G., 2007. Constipation and palliative care – where are we now? Int. J. Palliat. Nurs. 13 (1), 6–16.

Larkin, P., Sykes, N.P., Centeno, C., et al., 2008. The management of constipation in palliative care: clinical practice recommendations. Palliat. Med. 22, 796–807.

Nancekivell-Smith, R., 2010. Assessment and management of constipation in terminal disease. End of Life Care 4 (3), 56–63.

Points to consider

Don't assume that patients and their relatives know the link between opioids and constipation. Many patients need to have the link clearly explained to ensure that a laxative is taken regularly. Remember that prevention of constipation is much better for a patient than managing discomfort and pain associated with constipation. Also, when assessing a patient with advancing metastatic disease who has constipation, always consider the possibility of a spinal cord compression.

 Activity

> **Transitions and distress**
>
> Michelle is experiencing some major changes to her body and ability to perform her normal activities of daily living. Transition through the advancing stages of disease can be a frightening and anxious process for both Michelle and Simon.
>
> Under each of Michelle's symptoms, list what might be adding to her distress. Refer back to page 35 where we introduced the distress thermometer. Use this tool to assess what might be distressing Michelle.
>
> Now do some mind mapping: on a plain sheet of paper, write Michelle's name in the centre and then arrange all the symptoms she is experiencing around the edge. Include her distress and the needs of her family. Using a different coloured pen, write down an aspect of care that might be offered next to every symptom to help reduce her distress.
>
> NMC Domain 2: 2.4; 4.5

Further reading

O'Connor, M., 2008. An uncertain journey: coping with transitions, survival and recurrence. In: Payne, S., Seymour, J., Ingleton, C. (Eds.), Palliative care nursing: principles and evidence for practice, second ed. Open University Press, Maidenhead.

Goodhead, A., 2008. The importance of the nursing role in spiritual care of patients. End of Life Care 2 (2), 34–37.

Points to consider

It is important to know what might be the cause of distress. For many people, it is having to cope with physical symptoms; for others, it will be worry about financial issues or other members of the family. Worry beyond the self is often referred to as existential suffering. Every patient is different and gathering information from a wide range of sources will help the care team to make an informed assessment as to what might be causing the distress. Finding out how a person has managed a previously distressing situation can help in understanding how they respond to a current crisis. Previous experiences, even though the patient may have had a different diagnosis and symptoms, can be important when considering how to provide best care in distressing situations.

 Activity

> **Ongoing assessment**
>
> Using the EEMMA tool introduced on page 153, work through each of the stages to collate all the information we know about Michelle's current condition. This will help focus on planning care while keeping the approach holistic to the needs of both Michelle and her family.
>
> NMC Domain 3: 3.1; 3.3

Further reading

Steinhauser, K., Christakis, N., Clippe, E., 2000. Factors considered important at the end of life by patients, family, physicians and other care providers. J. Am. Med. Assoc. 284 (19), 2476–2482.

Points to consider

As symptoms become more complex and distressing, keeping a holistic focus of Michelle is essential in order to meet her needs and help to manage symptoms. Keeping Michelle central to the assessment is essential and the distress thermometer (see page 35) can help with this. Sometimes the complexity of symptoms a patient experiences can feel overwhelming, and separating out the problems, family needs and care interventions in this way can help focus on the many aspects that are often forgotten.

Case update

Michelle is started on dexamethasone for the spinal cord compression and a normal saline infusion to prepare her for treatment for the hypercalcaemia. After 3 days, Michelle continues to feel tired, though the vomiting is now settled and Michelle is enjoying small amounts of food. She particularly looks forward to the children visiting after school. Michelle is no longer constipated and continues to take regular laxatives. Michelle has been referred to the hospital Macmillan team for specialist management advice and support. The assessment unit team are now considering discharging Michelle home in the next few days.

Activity

Complex discharge

In considering Michelle going home, we are starting to make plans for a complex discharge. This needs to be planned carefully ensuring Michelle and her family's needs remain central to the decision-making process.

List what the challenges might be in planning this discharge.

Use the Roper, Logan and Tierney assessment tool introduced on page 130 to go through all of Michelle's holistic needs and start to think about what needs to be arranged for a successful discharge.

For example, consider the following:

- Support for Simon who is tired and missing work.
- Support for the children.
- Additional nursing care needed and involvement of community teams. Some of the services that might be available to the family are a night care service, for example Marie Curie Cancer Care, or a local hospice. Find out what is available in your local area.

Make a list of the practitioners who might be involved in discharge planning. Go back to the list of roles you were introduced to in Chapter 7.

NMC Domain 1:1.1; 1.2; 1.4; 1.5
NMC Domain 2: 2.1; 2.2; 2.4
NMC Domain 3: 3.1; 3.3; 3.8
NMC Domain 4: 4.6; 4.7

Further reading

Nunn, C., 2009. Facilitating a complex discharge from an acute hospital to home. End of Life Care 3 (3), 52–59.

Points to consider

In the Chapter 16, we explored the importance of knowing what the patient's priorities of care are and giving them choices about their care. When planning the discharge of a person with advancing disease, it is important to keep their needs central to the discharge process. It is important to consider the wider team working and ensure the discharge is planned in a safe and appropriate way. The above article focuses on the discharge of a woman with advanced multiple sclerosis, giving you ideas of how skills and knowledge can be transferred across disease pathways.

Case update

Michelle has told nursing staff that she is frightened at the thought of going home but doesn't want to upset Simon and the children who seem so excited. Staff have noticed her requesting analgesia more frequently for her abdominal pain and sleeping through the children's tea time visits. Simon has spoken independently to the care team about his anxiety at the plan for Michelle to go home.

Points to consider

Careful planning at this stage is vital and Simon needs to be kept central to the plans. Consideration needs to be given to how he is feeling about the proposed discharge and if he recognises how unwell Michelle now is. Sometimes a patient being discharged can be mistaken by family members as the person being 'well enough to go home'.

The next chapter explores the care Michelle and her family will need as she moves into the last days of her life.

Websites

The National End of Life Care Programme Website has up-to-date information and publications on all aspects of end of life care and is a good starting point to search for local and national publications, policies and ways of working: http://www .endoflifecareforadults. nhs.uk/ (accessed May 2011)

healthtalkonline is a charity-run Website that shares patients' experiences by facilitating them to tell their own story – many of these stories are presented in short film clips of 1–2 minutes. You can choose from a variety of headings including receiving bad news, cancer, and dying and bereavement: http://www. healthtalkonline.org/ (accessed May 2011).

23 Last days of life

Case update

Michelle is becoming increasingly sleepy and less responsive. The staff on duty at night time report that she is restless and appears frightened when Simon has gone home. After discussing this with Simon, he arranges for a friend to stay with the children at home and he spends the next few nights with her to help her settle. It has been decided at a team review to offer Michelle and Simon a bed on the specialist palliative care ward. Simon is taken to look at the ward by the Macmillan nurse and feels it is the right place for Michelle. It has a separate room where he can sleep and the children can play. He is hoping that once she is more settled, she may be able to go home. Michelle is very frightened at what is happening and finding it difficult to make any decisions.

 Activity

Terminal agitation

Consider how Michelle's fear may be addressed. What might be causing this fear?

List all the nursing care interventions that can support a person who is distressed in the last days of life. You might want to refer back to chapter 16 where we looked at spiritual and emotional distress and terminal agitation in the last days of life. Also reflect back to a patient you might have looked after on a previous placement who was distressed. Make a list of the care interventions that helped in this situation and then consider if they would be appropriate in Michelle's care.

NMC Domain 1: 1.1; 1.2
NMC Domain 2: 2.1; 2.3; 2.4; 2.5
NMC Domain 3: 3.1; 3.2; 3.3; 3.6; 3.7

Further reading

Forbes, C., 2007. Management of terminal delirium: a literature review and case study. Journal of Community Nursing 21 (4), 4–9.

Kyle, G., 2009. Terminal restlessness: causes, assessment and management. End of Life Care 3 (3), 8–12.

Namba, M., Morita, T., Imura, C., et al., 2007. Terminal delirium: families' experience. Palliat. Med. 21, 587–594.

Points to consider

The management of terminal agitation is an important part of managing last days of life. The way a person dies can have a big impact not only on relatives but also other patients and the care team.

 Activity

Psychological and spiritual support

Consider the support Simon will need. Who might be the best person to provide this?

Refer back to Chapter 7 where you were introduced to a range of roles within cancer services. Use this list to pick out who might be able to offer Simon support. Find out if the specialist palliative care ward/unit at your local hospital has any leaflets or information sheets that can be given to relatives. Reading through this information is a good way of being able to answer questions and offer support at the appropriate time. Consider how the information about Michelle being a 'lapsed catholic' might help in the ways distress might be managed.

NMC Domain 1: 1.1; 1.2; 1.5; 1.6
NMC Domain 2: 2.1; 2.4; 2.5
NMC Domain 3: 3.1; 3.3; 3.7; 3.9
NMC Domain 4: 4.4; 4.7

Further reading

Borg, L., Noble, H., 2010. Psychological issues associated with end stage cancer patients. End of Life Care 4 (2), 8–12.

Byrne, M., 2008. Spirituality in palliative care: what language do we need? Int. J. Palliat. Nurs. 14 (6), 274–280.

Royal College of Nursing, 2010. Spirituality in nursing care. Online. Available at: http://www.endoflifecareforadults.nhs.uk/publications/spirituality-in-nursing-care (accessed May 2011).

Points to consider

Throughout Michelle's diagnosis, she and Simon have made decisions together, so this is going to be a particularly difficult and lonely time for Simon to make decisions on his own. Sometimes the offer to sit with someone quietly can be a great sense of support and reassurance. Giving information clearly and sensitively will help the right decisions to be made. Leaflets can often answer simple questions quickly. At times of distress, information given is not always remembered so leaflets can be useful for a person to refer back to at a later date.

Case update

The following day, Michelle is transferred to the specialist palliative care ward where it has been agreed by the care team that Michelle is now moving into the last days of her life. The consultant agrees with the nursing staff and, after discussions with Simon, the Liverpool Care Pathway (LCP) is started. Her pain and anxiety will be managed by setting up a syringe driver since Michelle is no longer able to swallow her medication. This driver is effective in managing her pain and distress.

Activity

Using the Liverpool Care Pathway

Go to the Liverpool Care Pathway proforma found on the following Website:
http://www.liv.ac.uk/mcpcil/liverpool-care-pathway/ (accessed May 2011).

Complete the assessment of Michelle's current condition using the information you already have. As part of this assessment, you will be considering Michelle's spiritual and psychological needs, as well as the needs of Simon and other family members.

Make a list of what you need to consider when assessing her spiritual needs. From the admission documentation, you are aware that Michelle is a lapsed Catholic. Consider how you might address this with (a) Michelle and (b) Simon.

Now refer back to page 129 where we explored the concept of 'assessment'. Using a blank Roper, Logan and Tierney assessment tool, map out how Michelle's deteriorating condition will impact on each of her activities of living and list the nursing interventions that can assist in her holistic care to achieve comfort and maintain dignity.

NMC Domain 1: 1.1; 1.2; 1.5; 1.6
NMC Domain 2: 2.1; 2.2; 2.4; 2.5
NMC Domain 3: 3.1; 3.2; 3.7; 3.9
NMC Domain 4: 4.3; 4.6

Further reading

Go back to the above Website and select a last days of life care pathway for a specific disease group to read up on. This is a good resource to be familiar with when you are caring for people on non-cancer pathways.

Points to consider

Remember that religious need does not mean spiritual need. Always make a spiritual assessment ensuring the patient is assessed as a whole person. Religious need is just one of the aspects of care that may be important. Remember that every person has spiritual needs. Although a patient might not be practising the religion of their upbringing, it is important to be aware of this information. In this situation, it is worth having a conversation with Michelle and Simon to see if either of them want to speak with a chaplain or priest. It may be important to be aware that her parents or sister may require the support of a priest.

Case update

Six days later, Michelle dies peacefully with Simon and her children present. Michelle's parents and sister arrived at the ward 2 days previously and have been helping Simon with the children.

Activity

Care at the time of death

Consider the immediate actions that need to be taken now Michelle has died. What are the important things you know about Michelle that you are going to consider? Make a list of these.

You are aware Michelle is a lapsed Catholic. If you are not familiar with the rituals around dying and death for a person practising as a Catholic, look up on the Ethnicity Online Website:

http://www.ethnicityonline.net/ (accessed May 2011).

Note down any specific rituals that will be important before, at and after death. How do you feel at the thought of performing the last offices? What do you know about Michelle that will be important for whoever does this role?

NMC Domain 1: 1.1; 1.3
NMC Domain 2: 2.4; 2.5
NMC Domain 3: 3.4; 3.9

Further reading

National End of Life Care Programme guidance for staff responsible for care after death, http://www.endoflifecareforadults.nhs.uk/publications/guidance-for-staff-responsible-for-care-after-death (accessed May 2011).

Points to consider

Privacy and dignity are of vital importance both for Michelle and her grieving family. It is important that family and friends feel safe to express their grief and given the time they need to spend with Michelle. The hospital chaplain is there to support staff as much as patients and you might want one to come to the ward to offer support to you and your team.

 Activity

Care of self

You have cared for Michelle since she received her diagnosis in the outpatient clinic many months ago and have got to know her and her family well. Now make a list of the things you can do to support yourself and the other members of your team.

NMC Domain 1: 1.8
NMC Domain 2: 2.5; 2.6
NMC Domain 4: 4.4; 4.6

Further reading

Costello, J., 2011. Talking about death, dying and the end of life. Int. J. Palliat. Nurs. 17 (4), 15.

Cooper, J., Barrett, M., 2005. Aspects of caring for dying patients which cause anxiety to first year student nurses. Int. J. Palliat. Nurs. 11 (8), 423–430.

Points to consider

You are not on your own with difficult feelings. We can all get emotionally attached and upset when a patient dies. This is not a sign of weakness and other member of the care team can provide valuable support both during the process and afterwards. Don't forget the treat sheet you were introduced to on page 170. It can help to break the cycle of feeling upset about a patient or situation.

The final chapter in this case study takes Michelle on a completely different pathway. It is 5 years since Michelle was diagnosed and completed acute treatment for breast cancer. She has no evidence of cancer and has been attending follow-up care as an outpatient. She is now due to be discharged from the acute cancer setting. We explore the long-term effects of cancer and its treatment during the extended survivorship phase.

Websites

The National End of Life Care Programme Website has up-to-date information and publications on all aspects of end of life care and is a good starting point to search for local and national publications, policies and ways of working: http://www.endoflifecareforadults.nhs.uk/ (accessed May 2011).

healthtalkonline is a charity-run Website that shares patients' experiences by facilitating them to tell their own story – many of these stories are presented in short film clips of 1–2 minutes. You can choose from a variety of headings including receiving bad news, cancer, and dying and bereavement: http://www.healthtalkonline.org/ (accessed May 2011).

St Christopher's Hospice in London publishes *End of Life Care* four times per year. This is a journal for nurses who want to deliver best care to dying people at home, in care homes or in hospital: http://www.stchristophers.org.uk/ (accessed May 2011).

The National Council for Palliative Care is an umbrella organisation in England, Wales and Northern Ireland involved in all aspects of palliative and end of life care. It has a range of publications, news updates and views from the government, public and professional groups: http://www.ncpc.org.uk/ (accessed May 2011).

24 Living with and beyond cancer

Case update

It is now 5 years later and Michelle is 50 years old. She remains disease free and is about to be discharged from the follow-up clinic. She will be invited to have a mammography every 3 years as part of the national breast cancer screening programme.

From a medical point of view, Michelle has physically 'recovered' from her cancer and its treatment, however she is experiencing a number of chronic effects of treatment. Although Michelle's cytotoxic therapy did not induce an early menopause, she has experienced hot flushes, vaginal dryness, poor libido and weight gain since commencing tamoxifen.

The surgery has restricted her left arm and shoulder movement which has made carrying bags, swimming and household chores very difficult. Michelle is considering whether she should have a breast reconstruction. She feels that this may have a positive affect on her body image, although she is worried about undergoing further surgery.

The radiotherapy has resulted in dilated blood vessels under the skin around the mastectomy site. This is not painful but, visually, Michelle feels very conscious of this.

Any slight twinge, ache or pain Michelle experiences, she wonders if the cancer has come back. Michelle constantly fears the cancer may reoccur – this is quite debilitating and is a particular problem during the night, affecting her sleep. She is also concerned that the cancer might be linked genetically (even though she has no family history herself), and is anxious that her daughter may be at increased risk of developing breast cancer.

Michelle has been back at work for 4 years and, although she likes the people she works with, she is feeling bored and would like a new job that would stretch her mentally and have more potential to earn more money. She isn't sure whether she should tell prospective employers about her past medical history and is worried that if she moves jobs she may loss her entitlement to sick leave and pay.

Points to consider

It is incredibly daunting to no longer be seen by the consultant. Patients often express that they feel highly anxious about who will monitor them, in case of recurrent disease, feeling the responsibility of detecting recurrence is on them. For some patients, the fear of recurrence may diminish over time, but for many people, it affects their day-to-day lives. This is just one of the many uncertainties individuals have to deal with after cancer.

The role of the primary care team is paramount in supporting patients once they have been discharged from specialist care in the transition from being 'a cancer patient' into 'normal' life. However, patients never return to 'normal' – their lives are changed forever, whether it is a change of their physical function or appearance or the psychological fear of recurrence or loss of social role and economic status if the individual is unable to return to their pre-cancer employment. The severity and scope of the impact of cancer and its treatment will depend on many variables, but the long-term impact on the individual and their friends and family is enormous. Life will never be the same.

Because historically cancer survival rates have been so poor, there has been a lack of focus on how best to support individuals beyond diagnosis and treatment. With the increasing number of cancer survivors and the chronic nature of the disease, this has begun to change and the National Cancer Survivorship Initiative (Department of Health et al 2010) is focused on possible ways of supporting and prompting self-care in these individuals, as well as the research needed to identify the true extent of the long-term implications of cancer on individuals and society.

As a cancer survivor and a clinician, Mullan (1985:273) summarises: 'We can no longer save people from drowning [and then] leave them on the dock to cough and splutter on their own, in the belief we have performed all we can'.

References

Department of Health, Macmillan Cancer Support and NHS Improvements, 2010. National Cancer Survivorship Initiative: vision. HMSO, London.

 Activity

Living with and beyond cancer

What might Michelle's concerns be regarding being discharged from specialist care completely? What information should Michelle receive on her discharge?

Make a list of what the late effects of breast cancer surgery, radiotherapy, cytotoxic and endocrine therapy might be? What health promotion/education should Michelle receive to stay well in the future?

Find out about the known genetic inherited breast cancer conditions. Explore how knowing about carrying a defected gene that *may* cause cancer may affect an individual and their blood relatives. What might the ethical issues be relating to this area?

What signs and symptoms of recurrent breast cancer should Michelle be aware of? What might be other signs and symptoms for other types of cancers?

What discussion should have with healthcare professionals have with Michelle regarding her breast reconstruction? Find out what types of reconstructive surgery there are. What are the risks and the possible cosmetic effects that might result?

Watch the Institute of Medicine 'Lost in transition' video on YouTube:

http://www.youtube.com/watch?v=YhuqWM3dNAw (accessed May 2011).

NMC Domain 1: 1.2;1.3; 1.4
NMC Domain 2: 2.2; 2.3; 2.4; 2.5; 2.6
NMC Domain 3: 3.1; 3.2; 3.3; 3.4;
3.5; 3.7; 3.8;3.9; 3.10
NMC Domain 4: 4.1; 4.2

Mullan, F., 1985. Seasons of survival: reflections of a physician with cancer. New England Journal of Medicine 313, 270–273.

Further reading

Office for National Statistics, 2007. Survival rates in England, patients diagnosed 2001–2006. ONS, London.

Rachet, B., Maringe, C., Nur, U., et al., 2009. Population-based cancer survival trends in England and Wales up to 2007: an assessment of the NHS cancer plan for England. Lancet Oncol. 10 (4), 351–369.

25 Transferable skills for future placements

CHAPTER AIMS

- To reflect on core nursing skills
- To understand how to transfer skills and learning to other clinical areas
- To plan for future professional practice

Introduction

This book has explored a wide range of issues around caring for a patient with a cancer diagnosis. This chapter helps you to think about how you can transfer and consolidate your learning, knowledge and skills into other clinical placements, as well as a being a foundation for your ongoing professional nursing practice.

The knowledge, skills and experience you have gained while on your cancer/palliative care placement will be invaluable in your future practice, enabling you to care for patients in many diverse care settings. For instance, you may be caring for a patient on a cardiac ward who is experiencing cardiac arrhythmias, as a result of anthracycline cytotoxic therapy which was given 10 years previously for breast cancer. Alternatively, you may care for a patient on a surgical ward who is undergoing routine investigative surgery. As a result of the surgery, this patient may be diagnosed with cancer.

However, not all patients you will care for will have cancer, yet the core knowledge and skills (including essential skills clusters) you have developed through this practice placement can be transferred to every area of nursing.

Reflecting on core nursing skills

During your cancer/palliative care placement, you may have learned, developed and demonstrated many of the clinical skills which meet the NMC standards of competence for pre-registration education (NMC 2010). The following activities highlight some of these core skills and encourage you to reflect upon your current practice abilities. The activities focus on patients with other medical conditions/heath problems to help you transfer your knowledge and skills into other clinical situations and fields of practice.

Each of you will respond to each activity in your own way and at a different level, depending on the stage of your course and your individual abilities, development and progress. You should discuss these activities with your mentor or personal tutor, using your practice document to help you identify your achievements, demonstrate your competency and highlight any learning needs and opportunities. Your mentor may find these exercises helpful to guide you and support your learning.

 Activity

Essential skills clusters

What do you consider are the important issues when caring for a patient with a cancer diagnosis. Make a list of the core nursing skills needed to care for a patient with cancer and identify which part of the cancer pathway each skill might relate to.

Now consider which of the skills in your list might be important for care of a patient without a cancer diagnosis. What are the differences in your lists?

Refer to the NMC essential skills clusters (ESCs) (NMC 2010) in Box 25.1. Consider the ESCs you may have achieved while on your cancer/palliative care placement. How might you adapt these skills in other healthcare settings and with patients who do not have a cancer diagnosis? There may not be many differences.

NMC Domain 1: 1.1; 1.8
NMC Domain 4: 4.3; 4.4; 4.5

Box 25.1 ESC checklist

- Measures of height, weight, body mass index (BMI)
- Fluid balance
- Aseptic technique
- Dietary intake
- Medicines calculation
- Measurement and recording of temperature, pulse, respirations and blood pressure
- Medicine administration
- Intravenous fluids
- Enteral feeding
- Patient group directions
- Nutritional assessment
- Dehydration

Box 25.2 Documentation checklist

Review your practice documentation to reflect on all of the clinical skills you have achieved and those that still need to be assessed. Discuss these with your mentor to develop an action plan, ensuring that you are prepared for your next placement. If this is your final placement, your sign off mentor will be reviewing your achievements and assessing your overall performance.

The following activities explore some of the fundamental aspects that you need to consider when caring for patients to ensure you are providing up-to-date, relevant and comprehensive patient-centred care, while safeguarding vulnerable individuals.

Whatever stage you are at in your nursing education and irrespective of the healthcare setting, you are accountable for your actions and omissions and must work within the professional boundaries set out by the NMC (2008). As an accountable practitioner, you are accountable to the professional

governing body (the NMC), your employer, the law and yourself. Think about how your responses to the questions above link to the key aspects or pillars of accountability which include:

- professional
- legal
- employment
- ethical.

Activity

Accountability

You are preparing to discharge a widowed man you have looked after for 2 weeks on a surgical gastrointestinal ward. He has had a colostomy performed for benign bowel disease. The colostomy may be reversed in the future, but this decision will not be made by the medical team for several months. You might wish to consider reading a surgical book explaining the nature of the surgery he has had and the possible outcomes (such as Chapter 17 in Pudner 2010).

You are having a conversation with him about his discharge and he raises a few issues. Consider how you might respond to each of his questions and how your responses relate to your professional practice:

■ He asks you to explain his new flange and colostomy bag the stoma nurse has provided. This is a system you are not familiar with.

■ He asks that you leave out some of the information about his admission on the discharge letter since he does not want his daughter to know about his disease.

■ He asks that the community nurse who was looking after him before admission is not asked to go back to him since they did not see 'eye to eye'.

■ He asks you to reassure him that he will soon be back to 'normal'.

■ He is worried about being lonely when he gets home and asks if you will visit him.

NMC Domain 1: 1.1; 1.7; 1.8
NMC Domain 2: 2.5; 2.8
NMC Domain 3: 3.8
NMC Domain 4: 4.4

Refresh your understanding of the underpinning background of accountable practice by reading Chapter 1 in Caulfield (2005). You should refer back to Chapter 5 to revisit the ethical principles. Develop your responses further using this additional reading to help you justify your decisions.

Box 25.3 Professional practice checklist

■ Identify key healthcare professionals (within the healthcare setting and university) who you can discuss issues of your own accountable practice with.

■ Ensure that you have read up on and are aware of the current evidence regarding the nature of patient(s) conditions and care needs for those patients you are responsible for (alongside your mentor).

■ Reread the NMC code of conduct and refresh your understanding of your own personal and professional boundaries

■ You should discuss duty of care with your mentor and how this can be compromised and maintained.

■ If you have the opportunity, you may wish to visit a local coroners's court. Think about the role of the nurse in a particular case.

■ Ask your mentor how and what they are accountable for, with respect to their accountability to their employer.

Activity

Assessment

You are working on a surgical ward and preparing to assess the care needs of a man being admitted for planned (elective) surgery. While this might be your first experience of a surgical environment, you may have transferrable skills from your cancer placement. You have already picked up knowledge and skills about caring for a person with a cancer diagnosis and you can apply these experiences to the assessment process in this new environment.

Choose one of the nursing assessment tools you have been introduced to in your current placement or from this book (for example, the activities of living section on page 131, family assessment in Appendix two or pain assessment on page 137). Spend some time considering how the tool you have chosen might be used for a patient who has been admitted to an acute surgical environment for routine surgery and make some notes under each part of the assessment. To guide you with this activity, you might choose to look at some of the examples of surgical interventions given in the surgical placement pocket book in this series.

NMC Domain 3: 3.1; 3.3
NMC Domain 4: 4.1

Box 25.4 Principles of assessment checklist

1. Aims to gather information
2. Allows an opportunity to give information to the patient and family
3. Assists the patient to tell their own story
4. Ascertains patient understanding of what is planned for their care
5. Affirms patients' holistic identity and needs

Now refer back to your completed assessment tool for the surgical patient and check that you have covered these five principles.

For further information on the principles of assessment, refer to Chapter 1 in Holland et al (2008) which consolidates the principles of assessment as it is applies to the activities of living model.

Communication is a core skill that is central to effective high-quality health care. As well as communicating with patients and their carers, it is essential that we communicate with other healthcare professionals to ensure information is shared appropriately and in a timely fashion. It is important that we think about who we are communicating with; what the purpose of the communication is; what the person needs to know; what the best method of communication is; and when the best time to communicate is.

As well as preserving confidentiality in terms of professional accountability, patients have the legal right to confidentiality under the Data Protection Act 1998, the Human Rights Act 1998 and the common law duty of confidence (Freedom of Information Act 2000). They have the right to ask for a copy of their health records and any other personal information that healthcare organisations hold about them. Find out what the process is in your healthcare organisation in order for patients to access their medical records.

Activity

Communication

You are a final year student and preparing to hand over a critically ill woman to the nurses arriving on the next shift. The patient has been diagnosed with sepsis (see page 99) and is deteriorating. You have been caring for this patient for the past 4 days and have got to know her family quite well. Her husband has dementia.

Make notes on the important elements of what you need to communicate at this handover to the next shift under the following headings:

- Evaluation of current condition.
- Ongoing medical interventions.
- Role of multiprofessional team members.
- Evaluation of care delivered during the last shift.
- Ongoing observations and nursing care requirements (don't forget to consider her care needs from a holistic perspective. Refresh your memory on page 45).
- Relatives' understanding of the situation (go to page 32 to refresh your memory on supporting patients and relatives who may be given bad news).

You can refer back to page 99 where you were introduced to the principles of caring for a patient with sepsis. Use this as a checklist to review how you have planned your communication.

Read Jootun and McGhee G (2011) (see References) for guidance on communicating with a person who has a diagnosis of dementia. This will help to focus on the needs of the husband.

At every handover, there is the potential that vital information may not be communicated correctly and this can have a detrimental impact on the experiences and outcomes for the patient, relatives and care team. Therefore, you need to structure the way you communicate and be systematic in your approach to providing this information.

NMC Domain 1: 1.4; 1.5; 1.6
NMC Domain 2: 2.1; 2.2; 2.7; 2.8
NMC Domain 4: 4.3; 4.6

 Activity

Confidentiality

A man has been admitted to your ward without any family members with him. You have been asked to admit him and have completed a full assessment of his medical history, current health problems, care requirements and personal details using the hospital's admission documentation.

Consider your professional responsibility regarding the issue of confidentiality in the following situations:

- The doctor asks you what medications the patient is taking.
- You receive a phone call from a relative who wants to know how the patient is.

■ The ward waitress recognises the patient as a neighbour and asks you what is wrong with him.

■ The patient records office phones and ask you to confirm the patient's address.

Make some notes on how you would respond to each situation. What are the reasons for your answers? What are these based upon?

Almost all healthcare situations place patients in a vulnerable position and healthcare professionals have access to extremely personal and intimate patient information. As healthcare professionals, we have a legal and professional responsibility to safeguard verbal and written information. In addition, confidentiality is crucial to develop trusting relationships with patients.

NMC Domain 1: 1.1; 1.5; 1.6
NMC Domain 2: 2.1; 2.8

Now go back to your answers for the previous activity – Is there anything you would like to change? How might you act in future situations?

Think about possible or actual situations you may have encountered where information may have, or has, been disclosed. Remember, disclosure of information is only lawful and ethical if the individual has given consent to the information being passed on. Such consent must be freely and fully given. Revisit Chapter 8 which discusses consent.

To assist you to complete the confidentiality activity, it is invaluable to visit the NMC Website and reread the code of conduct (NMC 2008):

http://www.nmc-uk.org/Nurses-and-midwives/The-code/The-code-in-full/ (accessed May 2011).

Also, read the NMC advice on confidentiality (NMC 2009):

http://www.nmc-uk.org/Nurses-and-midwives/Advice-by-topic/A/Advice/Confidentiality/ (accessed May 2011).

In addition to these general guides, the NMC provides specific guidance for student nurses (NMC 2011) which will also aid your development:

http://www.nmc-uk.org/Documents/Guidance/Guidance-on-professional-conduct-for-nursing-and-midwifery-students.pdf (accessed May 2011).

Think about how this guidance helps student nurses make decisions regarding confidentiality. See Box 25.5 for some examples from the guidance that might help you complete this exercise.

Box 25.5 Examples from the NMC (2011) guidance on professional conduct for nursing and midwifery students

---

As a student nurse you should:

– respect a person's right to confidentiality

– not disclose information to anyone who is not entitled to it

– seek advice from your mentor or tutor before disclosing information if you believe someone may be at risk of harm

– follow the guidelines or policy on confidentiality as set out by your university and clinical placement provider

– be aware of and follow the NMC guidelines on confidentiality

Look up the Mental Capacity Act (2005) to explore possible situations where consent cannot be given:
http://www.legislation.gov.uk/ukpga/2005/9/contents (accessed May 2011).

Find out what should happen in situations where capacity is compromised in the healthcare setting.

 Activity

Decision making

A 15-year-old teenager with cystic fibrosis is admitted from his school to the medical assessment unit following an exacerbation of his respiratory condition. He is accompanied by his parents, who are keen for him to be transferred immediately to the respiratory ward for observation and treatment as an inpatient. However, he requests that he is treated quickly and allowed to go home and be seen by his cystic fibrosis specialist nurse as an outpatient.

In this exercise, you are encouraged to think about the ethical, legal and professional issues when considering his request. Make notes under each of the three headings to help you to explore the decision making:

1. Ethical: consider how you will balance doing good and doing no harm for all involved. To refresh your memory on ethical reasoning, turn to page 48.
2. Legal: what does the law say about a 15-year-old making a decision? What does the law say about the rights of parents of teenage children? More information is available at the NHS choices Website: http://www.nhs.uk/chq/Pages/900.aspx?CategoryID=62&SubCategoryID=66 (accessed May 2011).
3. Professional: what is your responsibility on decision making? Look at the NMC Website about professional responsibility in decision making: http://www.nmc-uk.org/Nurses-and-midwives/The-code/The-code-in-full/ (accessed May 2011).

NMC Domain 1: 1.1; 1.2; 1.3
NMC Domain 2: 2.1; 2.2; 2.3; 2.5
NMC Domain 3: 3.1; 3.8; 3.; 3.10

Now you have explored each perspective, consider who might be involved in this decision and what your role might be in the decision-making process. Go back to Chapter 7 and make a list of all the professionals you think will be important in this decision-making process. Make a list of additional team members who you may need to add to the list.

Help with decision making for children in transition can be found at the Association of Children's Palliative Care (Together for short lives) available at:http://www.act.org.uk/ (accessed May 2011).

Teenagers are often cared for in adult clinical areas and, if assessed as competent, can take an active part in the decision-making process regarding their own care.

Using the information you have gathered, now consider how you will evaluate the care given in addition to this patient's current condition. To do this, go to page 153, where you were introduced to the EEMMA assessment tool, and make notes under each section. To refresh your memory on anatomy and physiology of the lungs, refer back to your lecture notes or recommended physiology textbooks. Remember, relating anatomy and physiology to the evaluation process is an important aspect of ongoing patient care.

Reflect on how using a structured assessment tool can help you to evaluate the care given. Make some notes about this activity and be prepared to discuss the links of assessing a patient and ongoing evaluation with your mentor.

 Activity

Evaluating care

You are looking after a woman admitted with chronic bronchitis who is experiencing an acute exacerbation of her condition. A chest infection is suspected and she is commencing on oxygen therapy and intravenous fluids and is due to start intravenous antibiotics. Towards the end of the shift, you notice she is becoming increasingly drowsy and has a reduced urine output. Using your assessment skills, consider the important factors in evaluating her changing health status. To help you with this exercise, consider:

- the observations you would need to do to assess the effectiveness of the oxygen therapy and intravenous fluids. Include what can be measured (e.g. pulse, respiration rate) as well as direct patient observation (e.g. position in bed/number of pillows)
- the impact of her changing condition on each of the activities of living
- where this information is recorded and how it is communicated to the care team
- members of the care team who will need to know about your ongoing evaluations

NMC Domain 1: 1.5
NMC Domain 2: 2.7
NMC Domain 3: 3.1; 3.2; 3.3
NMC Domain 4: 4.2

As well as ensuring that healthcare professionals are competent to undertake a clinical procedure or intervention, it is essential that the rationale for undertaking the task is considered and that the procedure is based on current, reliable and valid research. Therefore, you need to make sure that procedures you undertake are based on research and are not just a result of 'this is the way we have always done it'. When you encounter a procedure you are unfamiliar with, you should take time to read up on the background and the current guidance, to ensure you are approaching the procedure based on the most up-to-date evidence.

However, research is not always available or there may be conflicting research results which present clear recommendations for practice. The knowledge and the expert opinion of an experienced healthcare professional may also constitute 'evidence-based practice', although this is subjective and often difficult to quantify. Usually a combination of evidence is used to dictate how a procedure is undertaken, based on local and national policy guidelines as well as research.

Review the research evidence you have identified via the university database. How reliable and valid is this research? Does the research support the hospital trust procedure guidelines? Refer back to any lecture notes you have been given or have written yourself during a practical session on the topic. Does this research and theory support the information your mentor provided for you?

 Activity

Evidence-based practice

You are caring for a patient who has had a stroke. They have lost the ability to swallow and are at risk of aspiration (fluid/food entering the lungs). Therefore, the patient has had a percutaneous endoscopic gastrostomy (PEG) tube cited so they can receive nutrition safely. You may be asked to assist in setting up the patient's enteral feed. If you are unfamiliar with this device and procedure, your mentor might demonstrate the practical procedure and inform you that this is up to date and is based on research evidence. You would observe the procedure, making a note of the main aspects of care in your notebook.

Access the hospital trust database of clinical procedures and read the enteral feeding procedure guidelines.

Refer back to your essential skills clusters in your clinical skills booklet. Read and familiarise yourself with the enteral feeding skills cluster.

Access the university electronic database to verify any information your mentor has provided by searching for relevant articles and books on the anatomy and physiology of PEG tubes and the care required to manage a patient receiving enteral feeding.

NMC Domain 1 : 1.1; 1.8; 1.9
NMC Domain 3: 3.4
NMC Domain 4: 4.1; 4.2; 4.4; 4.5; 4.6

Make a plan of how you intend to integrate your new knowledge into your clinical practice. This may be done by writing a piece of evidence to add to your portfolio. You could write a reflection, using a reflective model such as the Driscoll (2007) model introduced in Appendix one which allows you to follow a structured reflective process to integrate the evidence base and will help you consolidate your learning. When and where possible, you should include any references to support your discussion.

 Activity

Leadership

Using the same scenario as in the previous activity which focuses on evidence-based practice, think about how you will integrate this newly acquired theory and evidence into your clinical practice and how will you share your knowledge with your mentor, practice colleagues and fellow students. The NMC (2008) stipulates that, as healthcare professionals, we must share our knowledge and experience to improve patient care. This can be done in many ways, both formally and informally.

NMC Domain 1: 1.1; 1.3; 1.4; 1.5; 1.6
NMC Domain 2: 2.1; 2.2; 2.3;
NMC Domain 4: 4.1; 4.3; 4.4; 4.6; 4.7

Discuss your portfolio evidence/reflection with your mentor and highlight any new knowledge and any research which either supports or challenges any procedures you have been shown. You need to take care to do this in a respectful, sensitive, non-threatening manner in order to clarify your mentor's rationale for undertaking the procedure in the way they have. You need to seek further information to find out why they may have contravened the research you have found. Caution is required as your mentor may be using their expert knowledge and experience to adapt the procedure within a specific context. Listening is a key element of assertiveness; it demonstrates respect for the other person's opinion. Other non-verbal skills will also be needed so think about how your body language can reduce an aggressive approach to a discussion.

It may be appropriate to write a separate reflective piece to explore how you find such a discussion with your mentor. Think about what skills you used to approach the topic in order to explore your mentor's opinion and provide feedback on your discovery of this evidence.

Assertiveness is a core attribute that all healthcare professionals need to develop and is essential for effective communication and team working. Remember, feedback is a two-way process – just as your mentor will be providing you with feedback on your progress and achievements, you can feedback new information and theory that may contribute to improved patient care.

It may be a good opportunity to contact your personal tutor to explore the clinical procedure as well as ascertaining how reliable the evidence you have acquired is before you approach your mentor.

Find out if your university offers assertiveness training to help you explore assertiveness and communication skills for handling situations on placement to increase personal effectiveness.

When you have examined the evidence base and had a discussion with your mentor and/or personal tutor, you should take the opportunity to share your new knowledge with your fellow students on placement. This can be done to a greater or lesser extent depending on your confidence and progression through your course.

 Activity

Giving significant news

In many clinical environments, this is referred to as 'significant news' and may not just be a life-limiting diagnosis for a wide range of reasons. You are observing a doctor informing an elderly woman that she cannot be discharged home. Instead, referral has been made for a social care assessment so she can be transferred to a local care home. This is a decision that has already been discussed with her sons. Consider why this might be 'bad news' for this patient and list the things that might distress her. Consider this decision from a holistic perspective and make notes under the following headings:

- Physical.
- Emotional.
- Spiritual.
- Social.

To do this activity, give some thought to the losses she may already have experienced and to future losses. Now consider how this news might be given sensitively.

Return to the East Midlands Cancer Network guidelines for breaking bad (significant) news introduced on page 32, available at:

http://www.eastmidlandscancernetwork.nhs.uk/_HealthProfessionals-ServiceImprovement-SupportiveandPalliativeCare-BreakingBadNews.aspx (accessed May 2011)

Make notes under each of the 11 headings. This will help you to prepare to give the news to this patient. Here is a reminder of some essential elements of breaking bad (significant) news:

- Preparation.
- Find out what is already known.
- Offer explanations.
- Encourage expression of feelings.

- Summarise the conversation.
- Plan of action.
- Communicate with others.

Reflect back to page 208 where Michelle receives bad/significant news of her changing condition and make a list of all the things that can represent 'bad news'.

For further reading on loss and transition, refer to the article by Trowel (2008) (see References). If you are unsure about completing this activity, reading this article first will give you some ideas about losses in society that are not associated with dying.

NMC Domain 1: 1.1; 1.2; 1.3; 1.4; 1.5; 1.6
NMC Domain 2: 2.1; 2.2; 2.3; 2.4; 2.5
NMC Domain 4: 4.7

 Activity

Holistic care

You are working on a busy ward for care of the older person. A man who has been an inpatient for several weeks appears to be withdrawn and reluctant to chat with other patients or look forward to his afternoon visitors. When you ask him how he is feeling, he reluctantly tells you he is a 'bit down in spirit'. Consider what he might mean by this phrase. Make notes on what might be impacting on how he is feeling. Identify what information might be needed to assess his holistic needs.

Now refer to page 45 where we looked at the concept of holistic care. Consider how you might respond to what this patient has said to you. What factors do you need to take into account? What assessment tools can you use to help assess his anxiety/distress? Return to the distress thermometer introduced on page 35 and make some notes about what might be impacting on this patient. What nursing interventions might help? Write down some sentences that you might use to initially respond to his comment. Now consider multiprofessional colleagues who might be able to support the needs of this man.

NMC Domain 1: 1.2; 1.3; 1.4; 1.5
NMC Domain 2: 2.1; 2.2; 2.3; 2.4; 2.5
NMC Domain 3: 3.3; 3.4; 3.7

Holistic care means a person is viewed as a whole and this includes physical, psychosocial emotional and spiritual needs. The activities of daily living (ADLs) effectively explore the holistic needs of a person, taking a systematic approach.

For further reading to link holistic care to the ADLs, refer to Appendix 4 in Holland et al (2008) (see References).

For further reading about the concept of meeting spiritual needs in nursing, refer McSherry et al (2004) (see References).

Activity

Infection control

Working in cancer services, you will be exposed to some very specific infection control risks. Each clinical setting will have infection control policies that will assist you to maintain a safe environment for yourself and for others.

You are nursing a woman who requires a wound dressing to be changed. You are aware that the lady is known to have methicillin-resistant *Staphylococcus aureus* (MRSA). You are unsure of what precautions you should take.

Find the infection control policies and procedures of your current/next placement and look up MRSA. Find out who the link person is with responsibility for supporting ward staff with infection control queries.

Refer back to your lecture notes on infection control procedures and policies and read Gould (2011) (see References).

Write a care plan for undertaking this dressing and discuss this with your mentor. Find out how to contact the infection control team. Think about the psychosocial impact of having MRSA on the patient and make some notes which will help you answer her and her family's questions.

Refer back to page 99 to refresh your knowledge on reducing infection risk for a person who has an increased risk of acquiring an infection.

Visit the NHS Choices Website and read up on the common signs and symptoms of MRSA:

http://www.nhs.uk/Conditions/MRSA/Pages/Symptoms.aspx (accessed May 2011).

NMC Domain 1: 1.1; 1.2; 1.4; 1.5; 1.7; 1.8; 1.9
NMC Domain 2: 2.1; 2.2; 2.3; 2.7; 2.8
NMC Domain 3: 3.1; 3.2; 3.6; 3.8

 Activity

Record keeping

Your mentor asks you to complete a discharge letter to the community nursing team referring a postoperative patient for subcutaneous anticoagulation (in order to reduce the risk of deep vein thrombosis (DVT) which may result from limited mobility postoperatively). You have only just met the patient today and are not very familiar with this individual care requirements. Write down all the ways of ensuring that important information documented is correct and up to date for the community team. What should you document in order to maintain continuity of care and patient safety once discharged? What are the issues of confidentiality when communicating with agencies outside the acute clinical setting?

Refer to the NMC record keeping guidelines to consolidate your practice and knowledge: http://www.nmc-uk.org/Documents/Guidance/nmcGuidanceRecordKeeping GuidanceforNursesandMidwives.pdf (accessed May 2011).

Think about the legal aspects of record keeping. Find out how your documentation may be used in the event of a complaint about care given to a patient or in a case involving the coroner.

Remember, all documentation needs to be dated, the time of writing noted and signed (plus countersigned while you are a student nurse) and you must print your name clearly. It needs to be factual, recounting events that have occurred or care that needs to be given, and naming all individuals that have been involved or need to be involved. Never abbreviate and always explain jargon or technical terms.

NMC Domain 1: 1.1; 1.5; 1.6; 1.7
NMC Domain 2: 2.2; 2.3; 2.7; 2.8
NMC Domain 3: 3.6; 3.9
NMC Domain 4: 4.3; 4.6; 4.7

 Activity

Risk assessment

There may be situations in *all* clinical environments that may place you, co-workers, patients and visitors at risk of harm. As a student and qualified nurse, you have a responsibility to be aware of the specific risks in the environment you are working in and should ensure an assessment of the environment is undertaken. In your cancer services placement, you will have learned about the risks associates with giving chemotherapy, the hazards associated with spillage of chemotherapy or contaminated body fluids and the hazards of radiation. Now consider you are working on a mental health ward and some body fluid has been spilt on the floor. How would you assess the risks? What are the underpinning principles of dealing with a spillage? How will you pass this information to your colleagues? Refer to page 73 to refresh your knowledge on the management of spillages.

Now make a list of responsibilities of the nursing team:

- To deal with the spillage.
- To ensure all team members know what to do if a spillage happens again in the future.
- To ensure equipment needed is stored in the clinical area.
- To complete required documentation.

NMC Domain 1: 1.5; 1.7
NMC Domain 2: 2.2
NMC Domain 3: 3.6
NMC Domain 4: 4.3; 4.6

Visit the National Institute of Health and Clinical Excellence Website to read about risk assessment:

http://www.nice.org.uk/aboutnice/whoweare/aboutthehda/hdapublications/

risk_assessment_at_work_practical_examples_in_the_nhs.jsp (accessed May 2011).

Visit the Health and Safety Executive Website at:

http://www.hse.gov.uk/ (accessed May 2011).

Activity

Team working

Reflect on a couple of patients you have cared for during your current placement. Refer back to Chapter 7 and make a list of all the members of the multiprofessional team you have worked alongside. What were the main contributions each of the different professionals made towards patient care and management? How did their role link with your role?

Are there any healthcare professionals in the list you have not worked with or had the opportunity to find out what their specific role is in this clinical setting? If so, consider what their role might be, and if you still do not understand their roles, discuss them with your mentor, making a note for future placements. This can help you to focus on finding out more about these roles on your next placement and it may be possible to arrange insight visits so that you can work alongside these specific individuals. It is vital that you understand the roles of each professional in order to respect the boundaries of each role and appreciate the function of individual team members. Remember, you will all be working towards a common goal – high-quality, patient-centred care.

Consider why team working, particularly multiprofessional team working, is needed in the healthcare environment. Think about how well the multiprofessional team worked together while you were on placement. What aided it and what hampered it?

Read Daly (2004) (see References) to consider some of the wider issues that influence the delivery of multiprofessional care.

You may have had the chance to learn alongside other students from other healthcare disciplines, such as medicine, physiotherapy, occupational therapy and social work, in the classroom or in the clinical setting. A number of universities have introduced and integrated interprofessional educational learning into the health curricula. Find out from your own university how interprofessional learning takes place locally.

Read Kelley et al (2009) (see References) and visit The University of Nottingham's Website to find out more how interprofessional learning can enhance team working and improve understanding of role and professional boundaries:

http://www.nottingham.ac.uk/ciel/index.aspx (accessed May 2011).

On this Website, you can explore the learning outcomes for interprofessional learning and you can view the 'values exchange' scenarios that are used to consider different professionals' viewpoints and values.

As well as working in a team with other healthcare professionals, you will have been working within a nursing team. Think about how the nursing team functioned on your placement. How well did they communicate, collaborate and support each another? What do you consider are the advantages of working in a team?

NMC Domain 1: 1.4; 1.5; 1.6
NMC Domain 4: 4.6; 4.7

Future professional practice

During your final interview with your mentor for this placement, you should present your portfolio of evidence alongside your ongoing record of achievement (ORA), demonstrating your clinical competence achieved on this placement, as required by the NMC (2010). During your interview, your mentor should provide comprehensive constructive feedback on your performance as a whole and specific feedback related to the objectives and goals you agreed at the start of your placement. You may not have achieved all of the NMC competencies this time, perhaps due to lack of evidence of your abilities or as a result of a lack of opportunities to develop these skills. Your mentor should help you identify the competencies not achieved and support you to develop an action plan for future placements.

Your university will have set two progression points during your course. You need to find out when these are to ensure you have reached the required level of competence at these two points in order for you to progress from one part of the programme to the next. Normally the first progression point is at the end of year 1 and the second progression point is at the end of year 2. To pass the second progression point, you will need to demonstrate that you are increasingly working independently and taking more responsibility for you own learning and practice.

If this is your final placement, your sign off mentor will assess your overall competence. They will carefully be scrutinising your ability to deliver safe, effective care in practice and apply your theoretical knowledge. Overall, they will be assessing your competency and fitness to practise and they will confirm that you have successfully achieved all of the NMC practice requirements. Refer to

Chapter 6 to revise the role of the sign off mentor.

Once you have had your ORA document signed by your mentor, you should arrange to meet with your personal tutor who will review your achievements and countersign the ORA.

Before you start your next placement, you should read your competency outcomes and essential skills clusters and make a note of what was outstanding from your previous placement and identify what your leaning outcomes will be on the next placement. This will help you to think about how you might be able to meet these learning outcomes to maximise your learning opportunities and achievements throughout the rest of your nursing training programme.

If this is your final placement, you will be nearing the completion of your course. Even though you might have achieved your competencies, you will still need to reflect on and identify your strengths and areas of professional development following your placement. Nursing is a profession that requires life-long learning to ensure that practitioners maintain up-to-date knowledge and skills and you have a professional responsibility to continually reflect on your performance and address your learning needs.

Before you start your first job, you will need to identify what your learning and development needs will be during your period of preceptorship. Preceptorship is where newly qualified registered nurses are offered support by a more experienced registered nurse (a preceptor) in the early stages following their initial registration. This will allow you to consolidate your knowledge and skills and develop confidence in your new role, but to optimise this you should be able to identify and develop your particular learning needs from the outset. This might include orientation to the ward environment, to learn and become familiar with new policies and procedures, or it may be specific, such as how to care for a patient with a particular complex medical condition.

You may, at a later date, wish to pursue formal education in the form of 'learning beyond registration (LBR)' or 'continuing professional development' (CPD). You should discuss this with your line manager and investigate the local university's post-registered education provision.

Final comments

This book aimed to help you actively engage in the cancer/palliative care practice placement across a diverse range of healthcare settings. You have been guided through the complex cancer pathway and experience, explored anatomy and physiology, treatments, toxicities, symptom management and holistic needs throughout. You have also been encouraged to consider the impact of a cancer diagnosis on the patient, family and professional caregivers and respond to emotional, spiritual, social, psychological and physical needs.

Throughout your cancer/palliative care placement, we hope you have reflected on your own feelings, beliefs, values and experiences surrounding cancer and have developed knowledge and skills required to care for patients with a diagnosis of cancer. This will help you manage often complex and distressing situations in any clinical setting and will help you to develop your professional identity, underpinning your professional practice.

We wish you well in your future nursing career and hope we have inspired you to explore cancer/palliative care nursing further!

References

Caulfield, H., 2005. Accountability. Wiley-Blackwell, Edinburgh.

Daly, G., 2004. Understanding the barriers to multiprofessional collaboration. Nursing Times 100 (9), 78.

Driscoll, J., 2007. Practising clinical supervision, second ed. Baillière Tindall, Edinburgh.

Gould, D., 2011. MRSA: implications for hospitals and nursing homes. Nursing Standard 25 (18), 47–56.

Holland, K., Jenkins, J., Solomon, J., Whittam, S., 2008. Applying the Roper–Logan–Tierney model in practice, 2nd ed. Churchill Livingstone, Edinburgh.

Jootun, D., McGhee, G., 2011. Effective communication with people who have dementia. Nursing Standard 25 (25), 40–46.

Kelley, A., Sharman, A., Coates, A., et al., 2009. Using interprofessional learning in practice to improve multidisciplinary working. Nursing Times 105, 43.

McSherry, W., Cash, K., Ross, L., 2004. Meaning of spirituality: implications for nursing. Journal of Clinical Nursing 13 (8), 934–941.

Nursing and Midwifery Council, 2008. The code: standards of conduct performance and ethics for nurses and midwives. NMC, London.

Nursing and Midwifery Council, 2009. Confidentiality. Online. Available at: http://www.nmc-uk.org/Nurses-and-midwives/Advice-by-topic/A/Advice/Confidentiality/ (accessed May 2011).

Nursing and Midwifery Council, 2010. Essential skills clusters and guidance for their use (guidance G7.1.5b). Final: standards for pre-registration nursing education – Annexe 3. NMC, London.

Nursing and Midwifery Council, 2011. Guidance on professional conduct for nursing and midwifery students. NMC, London.

Pudner, R., 2010. Nursing the surgical patient, 3rd ed. Baillière Tindall, Edinburgh.

Trowel, F., 2008. using a framework to help cope with loss and transition. End of Life Care 2 (2), 38–42.

Websites

Health and Safety Executive, http://www
.hse.gov.uk/ (accessed May 2011).
NHS Choices, http://www.nhs.uk
(accessed May 2011).
National Institute for Health and Clinical
Excellence, http://www.nice.org.uk
(accessed May 2011).
University of Nottingham Interprofessional
Education, http://www.nottingham.ac.uk/
ciel/index.aspx (accessed May 2011).

Appendix 1: Driscoll's (2000) model of reflection

What? Returning to the situation

- What is the purpose of returning to this situation?
- What exactly occurred?
- What did you see?
- What did you do?
- What was your reaction?
- What did other people do (e.g. colleague, patient, relative)?
- What do you see as key aspects of the situation?

So what? Understanding the context

- What were you feeling at the time?
- What are you feeling now? Are there any differences and, if so, why?
- What were the effects of what you did (or did not do)?
- What good emerged from the situation (e.g. for self, others)?
- What troubles you, if anything?
- What were your experiences in comparison to your colleagues?
- What are the main reasons for feeling differently from your colleagues?

Now what? Modifying future outcomes

- What are the implications for you?
- What needs to happen to alter the situation?
- What are you going to do about the situation?
- What happens if you decide not to alter anything?
- What might you do differently if faced with a similar situation again?
- What information do you need to face a similar situation again?
- What are your best ways of getting information about the situation should it arise again?

Appendix 2: Family assessment

PART 1 – ON ADMISSION

Patient's name: **Hospital No:**

The purpose of a Family Assessment is to help the Multidisciplinary Team (MDT) to get to know and build up a relationship with the patient's significant others. It should also help the MDT to highlight any specific needs, concerns or potential bereavement risk factors.

Each family is unique –
the following questions are a guide only and can be adapted accordingly.

1. GENERAL

a. What is your knowledge of the patient's diagnosis?

b. What is your knowledge of the patient's present condition?

c. How do you feel about the patient's illness? (Any specific worries or concerns?)

2a. FAMILY

a. How are you coping as a family?

b. Are there any dependent/disabled/elderly family members?

c. What network of support/help is currently available?

2b. CHILDREN/ADOLESCENTS

a. Relationship to the patient?

b. Nature of relationship (ie. close and caring, distant etc)

c. What is their knowledge/understanding of the current situation?

Continued

2b. Continued

d. What support is currently available?

e. Is school/college aware?

f. What additional support can we offer?

3. SPIRITUAL SUPPORT

a. Are there any beliefs or values which are important to you?

b. How may we further support you with this?

4. CONCERNS/ISSUES

a. Identify any other concerns/issues?

5. GENERAL COMMENTS, OBSERVATIONS OR CONCERNS OF THE ASSESSOR

Assessment provided by .... Relationship ....

Interviewer .... Date/Time ....

PART 2 – DETAILS OF DEATH

Patient: .... Consultant: ....

Hospital No: .... Macmillan Nurse: ....

Other professional involvement: Counsellor ☐ Chaplain ☐ Social Worker ☐ Other ☐

Date of death: .... Time of death: ....

1. How was the death perceived by significant others? (e.g. sudden, specific problems with symptom control, peaceful, feelings regarding length of terminal phase.)

2. Staff's perception of the death

3. Who was present at the death   Relationship to patient   Reaction to death
(e.g. tearful, shocked/numb composed)

a. ....
b. ....
c. ....
d. ....

4. Any factors which may contribute to a complicated grief reaction for any significant others (e.g. nature of relationship, other significant losses, known psychological illness.)

5. Nature of available support (e.g. family, friends, community, professional.)

6a. Please identify anyone who you feel may need ongoing support.

Continued

6b. Details of significant others:

Name:

Address:

Post code:

Telephone no:

Relationship:

Name:

Address:

Post code:

Telephone no:

Relationship:

Name:

Address:

Post code:

Telephone no:

Relationship:

Name:

Address:

Post code:

Telephone no:

Relationship:

Completed by:

Signature   *Printed name*

Designation: Date:

CASE CONFERENCE

1. Any other concerns not previously hilighted

2. Action to be taken:

a. Condolence letter ☐

b. Bereavement/Counselling team ☐

c. Macmillan Nurse. Name: ☐

d. Others. Name: Designation: ☐

Signature: Date:

Designation:

Index

Index

Index

Index

Index

Index

Index

Index